The Berserker's Gardens and Forests

Bjørn Schindler

ISBN: 9788230361115

DEDICATION

To my beloved Bonnie, Amelia, and Zuzanna - three extraordinary women who inspire me every day, I dedicate this book.

I invite you on this magical journey, where together we traverse the paths of our ancestors, discover secrets encrypted in plants, herbs, and algae, and draw from the wisdom contained in traditional medicine. In this expedition, full of learning and discoveries, we recognize the power and wisdom of nature, which provides us with harmony and health.

My love for you is like a mysterious forest, where every tree, every leaf, every tuft of moss has its own story and meaning. This book is like a map to that forest, filled with invitations to uncover and understand its mysteries.

May this book, written with love for you and for nature, serve you as a guide to health and harmony. In my heart, you are not only my family but also co-travelers, who add luster and meaning to this journey.

Thank you for being with me on this journey. The adventure begins here and now. With love, Your.. Bjørn

"Nature itself is the best physician." - Hippocrates

PROLOG

For many centuries, natural healing methods, regarded as artifacts of our ancestors, have successfully treated a variety of ailments. In the era of scientific and technological progress, at a time when man has conquered the moon, and the boundaries between the digital and the real world are becoming increasingly blurred, natural medicine is often discriminated against and neglected. How primitive it seems to use plants and herbs when our pharmacy shelves gleam with complex chemical formulas, antibiotics, pharmaceuticals designed to combat every disease we know.

However, when we look at reality, we see that despite enormous advances in medicine, lifestyle diseases such as diabetes, hypertension, obesity, and depression, are still with us. Even worse, their incidence is increasing, despite the use of the most efficient antibiotics and the most modern pharmaceuticals. Is this a sign that we are missing something important in our understanding of health and treatment?

In this book, we return to our roots, to wisdom passed down from generation to generation, where nature was our pharmacist. We will examine the power of plants that grew from the same earth as us. Nordic, Slavic, and Caucasian medicine, over centuries, has managed to identify and utilize nature's treasures in treating many ailments.

This knowledge, often neglected and marginalized in our era of antibiotics, synthetic drugs, and pharmaceuticals, deserves rediscovery and appreciation. It is our heritage, which has survived despite the currents of history, science, and culture. We are not proposing to abandon modern medicine in favor of a complete return to nature. Instead, we point to the importance of a holistic approach, which neatly integrates the best of both worlds.

Knowledge about herbs, their effects, and medicinal properties can serve as a powerful supplement to modern therapy, not as its direct competitor. Natural medicine is not only an ancient treasury of knowledge but also a reminder of the deep connection between us and nature, about harmony that we can so easily lose in the noise of everyday life. In an era when humanity struggles with the challenges of isolation from the natural world, an ever-faster pace of life, and increasing stress, understanding and utilizing the gifts of nature can be crucial not only for our physical health but also for our mental and spiritual health.

I would like to take you on a journey that will take you through ages, regions, and cultures, allowing you to discover forgotten traditions and herbal secrets. During this exciting journey, we will show you how to benefit from this ancient knowledge to improve your health, wellbeing, and even your quality of life. It is a journey not only to our shared past but also to our place in the natural world.

This is, above all, a journey to the future of medicine - a future that is more integrated, holistic, and respects the invaluable power of nature. Knowledge about herbs is our gift passed down through generations - it's time to utilize it again.

Viking Resurrection: Scandinavian Herbal Medicine and Gifts of Nature

„Health is the real wealth, not pieces of gold and silver. Nature is always the most beautiful backdrop for this wealth."
- Magatma Gandhi

The world of the Vikings is not only stories of bold warriors traversing the seas in search of new lands and treasures. It is also a story of quiet strength and wisdom, hidden in the Scandinavian forests, meadows, and coasts, which formed the basis of their health and prosperity.

In this part of our journey, we will immerse ourselves in the heritage of Nordic natural medicine, discovering the treasures that our ancestors long ago discovered and that can still serve us today.

The lands of Scandinavia, with its harsh climate, long winters, and short but intense summers, gave rise to plants that were able to survive and thrive in these conditions. This is the terrain where bright summer meets dark winter, where the sea meets the land, where harsh mountains meet fertile valleys.

This diversity of landscapes has produced a wealth of plants that the Vikings utilized in their everyday medicine. A variety of herbs, roots, berries, and mushrooms that grew in these lands formed the basis of Scandinavian herbalism. These natural products were not only consumed as food but also used to treat various ailments, from headaches to infections and chronic diseases. Through the following pages, you will discover the secrets of this ancient medicine, understand why the Vikings drew from the treasures of nature, and how we can apply this wisdom in modern times. We will discover the herbs that were crucial to the health of the Vikings, learn how to prepare and use them, and understand why natural medicine remains so important to contemporary Scandinavians.

So let's fasten our seatbelts, open our minds, and begin our journey back to Viking times, uncovering a medicine that has stood the test of time and whose power we can harness today.

So let's begin this magical journey where you will learn the secrets of nature, hidden in plants, herbs, and algae. These pages are your invitation to a world where medicine merges with tradition, and science with nature. Together, we will discover uncharted corners of our planet, immerse ourselves in dense forests, uncover the secrets of underwater gardens, and finally lose ourselves in the aromas and tastes of recipes that I have prepared especially for you.

Prepare for an exciting exploration, a journey full of adventure along the paths of our ancestors. Each page, each recipe, are steps on the staircase leading to a healthier and more harmonious life. So let's start this expedition, where at every step awaits learning, discovery, and above all, the pleasure of uncovering.

I'm glad you're with me.
Let's get started!

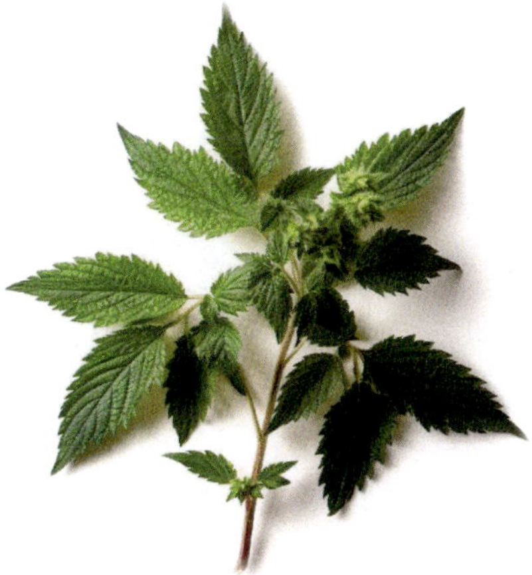

Stinging Nettle (Urtica dioica)
This common plant has powerful anti-inflammatory and detoxifying properties. It is also rich in vitamins and minerals, including iron, which is necessary for blood health.

Nettle Infusion

Ingredients:
- 1 tablespoon of dried nettle leaves (Urtica dioica)
- 1 cup of boiling water

Preparation: Collect fresh nettle leaves (remember to wear gloves to avoid being stung) and leave them to dry in the shade, in a well-ventilated place, until they become brittle. You can also use a ready-made, dried product available in herbal shops. Place the dried nettle leaves in a cup or teapot. Pour boiling water over the leaves and leave to infuse for about 10 minutes. Strain the infusion and leave to cool. You can add a tablespoon of honey or lemon for flavor, if you want.

Nutritional Richness: Nettle contains high amounts of many vitamins and minerals. It is particularly rich in vitamin A, key for eye health, as well as B vitamins, which aid in regulating metabolic functions and nervous system health. Additionally, nettle is a good source of vitamin C, which has strong antioxidant properties and supports the immune system. Of the minerals, nettle contains a lot of iron, which is necessary for blood health, as well as calcium, magnesium, manganese, phosphorus, and potassium.

Anti-inflammatory Properties: Nettle infusion is known for its anti-inflammatory properties, which can help alleviate symptoms of conditions such as arthritis, joint diseases, and other inflammatory states.

Detoxifying Properties: Nettle supports kidney function, aiding in the natural process of detoxifying the body from toxins. By drinking nettle infusion, we can support detoxification processes in our bodies.

Support for the Urinary System: Nettle is well-known for its diuretic properties. It aids in the removal of toxins from the body by stimulating the diuretic process. This has a positive effect on the kidneys and bladder, aiding in the treatment of urinary tract infections and preventing kidney stones.

Support for the Immune System: Thanks to its high content of vitamins A, C, and K, as well as many different minerals, nettle can help strengthen the immune system and assist the body in fighting off diseases.

Preventing Anemia: Nettle is rich in iron, which makes it excellent for people suffering from anemia and other disorders related to iron deficiency. Regular consumption of nettle can help in raising hemoglobin and red blood cell levels.

Joint Health Support: The anti-inflammatory properties of nettle can help alleviate symptoms of inflammatory joint conditions, such as rheumatoid arthritis.

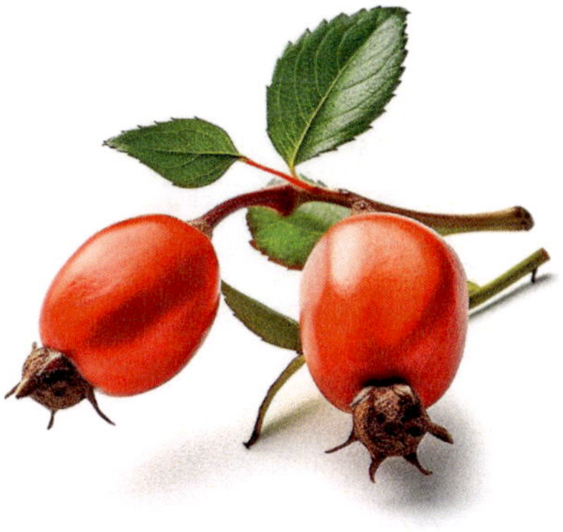

Wild Rose (Rosa canina)
The fruits of the wild rose, known as rose hips, are incredibly rich in vitamin C, making them a powerful support for the immune system. They also have anti-inflammatory and antibacterial properties.

Rosehip Infusion

Ingredients:
- 2 tablespoons dried wild rose fruits
- 2 cups boiling water

Preparation: Place the dried wild rose fruits in a cup or teapot. Pour the fruits with boiling water and let it steep for about 15-20 minutes. Strain the infusion and allow it to cool.
You can add a spoonful of honey for taste, if you want.

Rosenhip Syrup

Ingredients:
500 g wild rose fruits
1 liter of water 500 g of sugar (you can adjust the amount to taste)u)

Preparation: Wash the wild rose fruits, remove the stalks and seeds, then cover with water and simmer on low heat for about 1 hour until the fruits soften. Strain the fruits through a sieve or dense fabric, squeezing out as much juice as possible. Reheat the juice and add sugar, stirring until dissolved. Pour the syrup into sterile bottles or jars. Seal tightly.

High Vitamin C Content: The wild rose is one of the richest sources of vitamin C, a substance that plays a key role in many metabolic processes. Vitamin C is a potent antioxidant that helps protect the body from damage caused by free radicals, and also supports the immune system and collagen production, which is key for the health of skin, hair, nails, and joints.

Anti-Inflammatory Properties: The infusion made from wild rose fruits is known for its anti-inflammatory properties that can help relieve symptoms of inflammatory conditions such as osteoarthritis. Supports Digestive Health: Wild rose has purgative properties that can aid in regulating digestive functions, supporting both peristalsis and digestive processes.

Supports Skin Health: Thanks to its high vitamin C content and other antioxidants, the wild rose infusion can help protect the skin from damage caused by free radicals, promote collagen production, and support a healthy appearance of the skin.

Supports the Immune System: With its high vitamin C content and other nutrients, the wild rose is known for its immune-boosting properties.

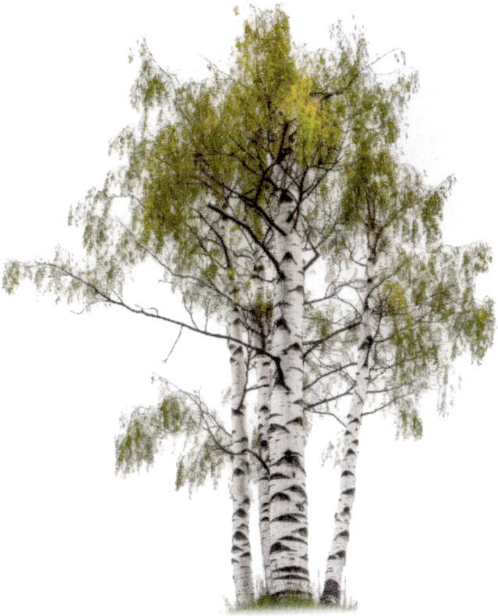

Birch (Betula)
Vikings made use of various parts of the birch tree - leaves, bark, and sap. Birch has diuretic, analgesic, and anti-inflammatory properties.

Birch Leaf Tea

Ingredients:
- 2 tablespoons of dried birch leaves
- 2 cups of boiling water

Preparation: Place the dried birch leaves in a cup or teapot. Pour boiling water over the leaves and let it steep for about 15-20 minutes. Strain the tea and let it cool. The tea can be served with honey.

Birch leaves are rich in flavonoids, which are powerful antioxidants, and also contain phenolic acid, which has anti-inflammatory and antibacterial properties. Birch leaf tea is often used to alleviate symptoms related to urinary tract inflammation and is also recommended as a natural diuretic that can aid kidney function and detoxify the body.

Birch Sap Syrup

Ingredients:
- 1 liter of birch sap
- 500 g of sugar or honey

Preparation: Heat the birch sap in a pot on low heat. When the sap starts to warm, add the sugar and stir until the sugar dissolves.

Simmer on low heat until the sap starts to thicken and attains the consistency of syrup. Pour the hot syrup into sterile bottles or jars and seal immediately.

Birch sap is a natural source of many nutrients, including vitamin C, potassium, magnesium, manganese, zinc, and folic acid. It is a natural detoxifying drink that helps cleanse the body and improve overall condition. Regular consumption of birch sap can contribute to the improved condition of skin, hair, and nails.

Birch Bark Infusion

Ingredients:
- 1 tablespoon of finely crushed birch bark
- 2 cups of boiling water

Preparation: Place the finely crushed birch bark in a cup. Pour boiling water over the bark and let it steep for about 20 minutes. Strain and let it cool. The infusion can be served with honey. Remember that birch bark should be collected responsibly and ethically, only from trees that are slated for logging or that have naturally shed pieces of bark. Living trees should never be harmed by stripping bark.

Birch bark contains compounds such as betulin and betulinol, which have strong anti-inflammatory, antibacterial, and anticancer properties. Birch bark infusions are often used to treat various skin conditions, such as eczema, psoriasis, and minor burns.

Additionally, birch bark has analgesic properties that can be helpful for headaches and muscle pains. All these health benefits make birch an extremely valuable resource in traditional medicine.

Flavonoids and Phenols: Birch leaves contain many flavonoids and phenolic compounds that act as powerful antioxidants. They help to neutralize harmful free radicals in the body, which can prevent chronic diseases like heart disease and certain forms of cancer.

Saponins: Birch leaves contain saponins, which have numerous health benefits, including the ability to lower cholesterol levels, improve immune system health, and aid in the treatment of some skin diseases.

Birch, also known as the „tree of life," is a highly prized ingredient in natural medicine and pharmaceuticals. It owes its reputation to its exceptional content of bioactive substances such as flavonoids, terpenoids, saponins, and polyphenols. In traditional Nordic medicine, birch leaves were used as a potent diuretic, helping to eliminate excess water and toxins from the body. The anti-inflammatory and antiseptic properties of birch bark were utilized in treating inflammatory skin conditions, ulcers, and other infections.

In modern pharmaceuticals, birch extract is increasingly utilized due to its potent anti-cancer properties. Studies show that betulin and betulinol, two bioactive substances present in birch bark, can inhibit the growth and development of cancer cells. Even birch sap, called „birch wine," is a rich source of minerals and vitamins, including vitamin C, potassium, and magnesium, and is often used as a natural strengthening and nourishing agent.

Thus, we see that birch is a true treasure trove of nature, whose secrets we continue to uncover. With each new study, each new discovery, birch reaffirms its status as an invaluable plant in natural medicine and pharmaceuticals.

Betulinic Acid: Birch bark is rich in betulinic acid, which has strong anti-inflammatory, antibacterial, and anti-cancer properties. Betulinic acid is being researched for its potential application in the treatment of certain forms of cancer, such as skin cancer.

Minerals: Birch sap is a natural source of many minerals, such as manganese, magnesium, calcium, zinc, potassium, and sodium. These minerals are essential for the proper functioning of many processes in the body, including bone health, the nervous system, and the cardiovascular system.

Vitamins: Birch sap is also a source of vitamin C, which the body needs to strengthen the immune system, produce collagen, and improve iron absorption.

For centuries, the birch tree, this symbol of purity and renewal, has not only served as a source of inspiration for poets and painters but also as a key ingredient in folk medicine and today's phytotherapy, providing valuable active substances contained in its leaves, bark, sap, and buds that help combat many ailments, from urinary tract infections to skin problems.

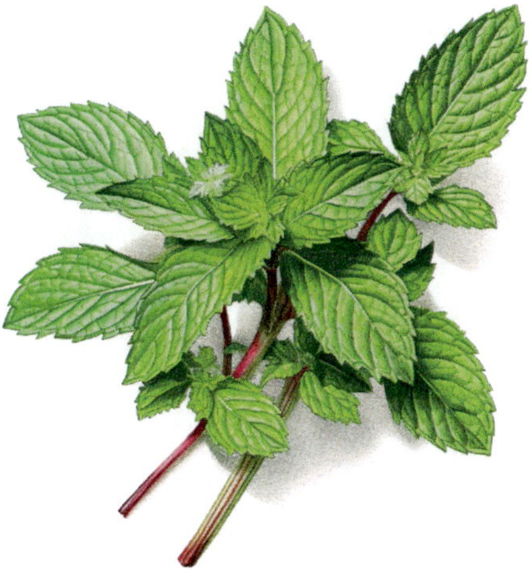

Peppermint (Mentha piperita)
A popular medicinal plant, peppermint is known for its properties that soothe the digestive system, aid digestion, and alleviate headaches.

Peppermint Infusion

Ingredients:
- 1 tablespoon fresh or dried peppermint leaves
- 1 cup boiling water

Preparation: Place the peppermint leaves in a cup. Pour over the boiling water and cover the cup. Allow to steep for about 10 minutes. Strain the infusion to remove the leaves..

The infusion can be served both hot and cold. If you wish, you can add a little honey for sweetness. Peppermint in the kitchen Peppermint can also be used in the kitchen to prepare various dishes and drinks. It can be added to salads, sauces, desserts, as well as cocktails and other beverages

Fresh Peppermint Leaves: Adding fresh peppermint leaves to lemonade or tea creates a refreshing drink, perfect for hot days.

Vitamins: Peppermint is a source of many vitamins, such as vitamins A and C, which are potent antioxidants. Vitamin A is necessary for eye and skin health, and vitamin C aids in the production of collagen and strengthens the immune system.

Minerals: Peppermint contains various minerals, such as magnesium, calcium, phosphorus, and potassium, which are essential for many bodily functions, such as bone health, proper functioning of the nervous system, and maintaining electrolyte balance.

Warming Ingredients: Essential oils, like menthol found in peppermint, have warming and analgesic effects. They can alleviate symptoms of colds and flu, such as sore throat, cough, and nasal congestion.

Antioxidants: Peppermint is rich in antioxidants, which help combat free radicals and may help prevent many chronic diseases, such as heart disease and cancer.

Antibacterial and Antiviral Components: The essential oils in peppermint also have antibacterial and antiviral properties, which can help fight off infections.

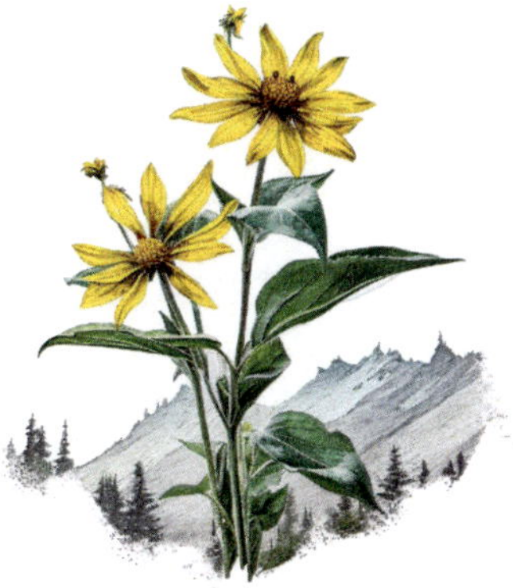

Mountain Arnica (Arnica montana)
Externally used, arnica is excellent for bruises, contusions, and swellings, thanks to its analgesic and anti-inflammatory properties.

Mountain arnica, also known as the „golden sun of the mountains", is another treasure of natural medicine, particularly appreciated by the ancient Vikings and other European peoples. This Alpine pearl was especially valued for its potent anti-inflammatory and analgesic properties. In traditional herbal medicine, mountain arnica was used externally in the form of ointments, liquids, or compresses for bruises, contusions, swellings, and even inflammatory skin conditions and ulcers. These properties are attributed to the presence of helenalin - a substance with confirmed anti-inflammatory and analgesic action. In modern pharmacy, arnica extract is often used as an ingredient in preparations used after injuries or surgical procedures, supporting the healing process and reducing swelling. Moreover, studies suggest the potential use of arnica in the therapy of certain heart diseases, thanks to its ability to dilate blood vessels.

However, it is worth emphasizing that despite its undeniable benefits, Mountain Arnica is a plant with strong effects, which can cause skin irritation or allergic reactions. Therefore, it should always be used in moderation and under the supervision of a specialist. This is another example of how nature's treasures can serve human health. Mountain Arnica, with its golden flowers and potent medicinal properties, deserves a special place in our herbal and pharmaceutical medicine.

Recipe for Ointment

Ingredients:
- 1 cup of coconut oil or olive oil
- 1/4 cup of dried arnica flowers
- 1/4 cup of beeswax

Preparation: Heat the oil in a pot over low heat. Add arnica flowers and simmer on low heat for at least 2 hours. Strain the mixture through a sieve to separate the flowers from the oil. Make sure all the oil is drained. In the same pot, melt the beeswax over low heat. When the wax is completely melted, add the arnica oil to it and mix thoroughly. Then quickly pour the mixture into clean jars or containers. Allow to cool.

How to use arnica ointment?
Arnica is used externally and is particularly effective in treating bruises, contusions, and swellings. The ointment should be applied directly to the area requiring treatment, avoiding open wounds or scars. It should not be applied to mucous membranes or open wounds as it can cause irritation. Remember that arnica is a herb that can cause allergic reactions in some people. It is always worth testing the ointment on a small area of skin before applying it to a larger area.

Sesquiterpene lactones: These are the active ingredients of arnica that have strong analgesic and anti-inflammatory action. The main sesquiterpene lactone in arnica is helenalin, which helps in treating inflammatory conditions and pain.

Flavonoids: Arnica contains various flavonoids, which are strong antioxidants. Antioxidants help to combat free radicals in the body that can lead to various chronic diseases.

Phenolic acids: These chemical compounds have antibacterial and antifungal effects. They help protect the body against various pathogens.

Essential oils: Arnica also contains essential oils, which have various health benefits, including anti-inflammatory and analgesic effects.

Mountain Arnica, also known as ,gold of the mountains', has been a valued herb in folk medicine and today's phytotherapy for centuries, especially for its strong anti-inflammatory and analgesic properties.

The application of this herb ranges from treating bruises, sprains, and contusions, to relieving muscle and joint pain, making it an invaluable element in a natural home medicine cabinet

If you notice any symptoms of irritation or allergic reaction, stop using the ointment and consult a doctor.

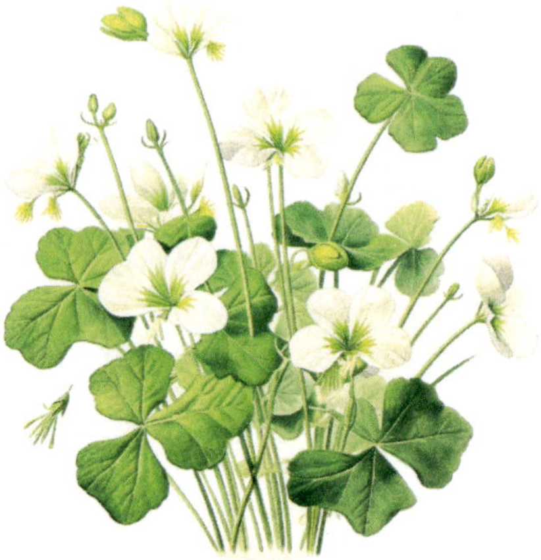

Wood Sorrel (Oxalis acetosella)
Wood Sorrel is a known source of Vitamin C.

It was also used as a purgative and a cleansing agent for the body. Wood Sorrel is a plant that is commonly found in the forest understory throughout Northern Europe. It is not only pretty but also edible and has many uses in natural medicine. Here are two examples of how you can use it

Wood Sorrel Salad

The young leaves of wood sorrel have a sour taste, which makes them an ideal addition to spring salads. You can simply wash, dry, and add them to the salad. The leaves are rich in Vitamin C, making them a gre-at addition to a meal.

Wood Sorrel Infusion

Wood sorrel can also be used to make tea. It's simple:

Ingredients:

- 1 tablespoon fresh wood sorrel leaves
- 1 cup boiling water

Preparation: Wash the wood sorrel leaves and place them in a jug or cup. Pour the leaves with boiling water and let it brew for about 10 minutes. Strain the drink and serve warm. A wood sorrel brew is not only tasty, but also has medicinal properties. It is diuretic and can help in the treatment of urinary tract infections. In addition, it has analgesic and antipyretic properties.

Vitamin C: This vitamin is a powerful antioxidant that helps protect the body from free radicals. Vitamin C also helps in the production of collagen, which is necessary for the health of skin, hair, and nails.

Oxalic acid: Wood sorrel contains oxalic acid, which is a natural antibacterial and antifungal agent. This helps to protect the body from various infections

Flavonoids: Wood sorrel also contains flavonoids, which are potent antioxidants. They help to fight free radicals in the body that can lead to various chronic diseases.

Minerals: Wood sorrel is also a source of various minerals, such as magnesium, potassium, and calcium, which are necessary for the healthy functioning of the body

Remember, while wood sorrel is edible and has many uses in natural medicine, it also contains oxalic acid, which can be harmful in large amounts.

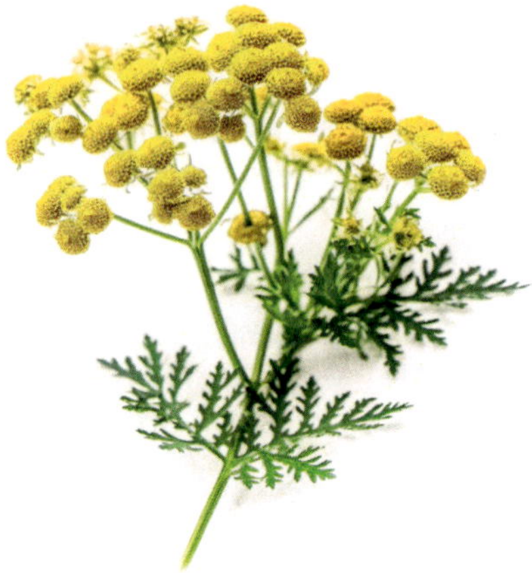

Common Tansy (Tanacetum vulgare)
Common Tansy, also known as the „mother of herbs," has a long history of use in folk medicine. Tansy was used in folk medicine for a whole range of ailments, from parasites to digestive disorders

Tansy Infusion

This infusion is often used in folk medicine to treat various ailments, such as digestive problems, parasites, and gynecological complaints.

Ingredients:

- 1 teaspoon of dried tansy leaves
- 1 cup of boiling water

Preparation: Place the dried tansy leaves in a jug or cup. Pour the leaves with boiling water and let it steep for about 10 minutes. Strain the infusion and drink it warm.

Tansy Ointment

Tansy ointment is often applied externally to the skin to alleviate ailments such as bruises, swelling, and inflammation.

Ingredients:

- 1 cup of dried tansy leaves
- 1 cup of coconut oil

Preparation: Place the tansy leaves and coconut oil in a pot and heat over low heat for about 2 hours. After 2 hours, strain the mixture and transfer it to a clean jar. Allow it to cool. Apply the prepared ointment to the skin as needed.

Flavonoids: These are powerful antioxidants that help fight free radicals in the body. They also help protect the heart and circulatory system.

Thujones: This is a component that helps in treating digestive problems, such as diarrhea and dyspepsia.

Tannic acid: This is a component that helps in treating digestive problems, such as diarrhea and dyspepsia.

Sesquiterpenes: Tansy contains sesquiterpenes, which show anti-inflammatory and analgesic action, making it effective in treating inflammatory conditions and pain.

Camphor and cineole: These components have antiseptic and antibacterial effects, making them effective in treating skin infections.

Tansy, also known as Tanacetum vulgare, was one of the basic plants used in natural medicine by the Vikings and ancient peoples of Europe. It was valued for its strong anti-inflammatory and antibacterial properties, which made it an invaluable ingredient in many medicines. The Vikings used tansy to combat skin ailments, insect bites, and even as an effective antiparasitic agent

In ancient Europe, tansy was also used as an analgesic and calming agent, as well as for treating stomach ailments. They believed that this versatile herbal remedy was a gift from the gods, capable of supporting health and wellbeing.

Common tansy, sometimes called „golden serpent" or „sun of the earth", is a plant that has long been regarded as a treasure of natural medicine, especially among the Vikings and other European peoples. Its exceptionally intense, golden flowers are not only beautiful but also full of medicinal properties. For centuries, tansy has been used as a natural remedy for various ailments. Its leaves and flowers contain a range of active ingredients, including flavonoids, essential oils, and sesquiterpenes, which have anti-inflammatory, antibacterial, antifungal, and even anti-cancer properties.

The Vikings used tansy to treat wounds, skin ailments, and also as an analgesic. Modern research confirms that tansy oil can effectively relieve pain, making it a valuable component of ointments and balms. But tansy is not only a medicine. Its intensely yellow flowers were used for dyeing fabrics, and the aromatic leaves were used to flavor beer and wine, testifying to the versatility of this plant. Today, even though tansy is often overlooked, its significance in natural medicine is undeniable. This golden plant, with its powerful medicinal properties and multifunctionality, deserves a special place in our herbal medicine cabinet.

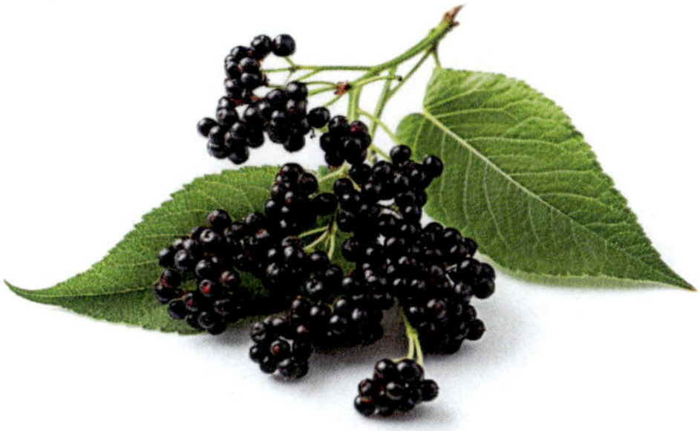

Black Elderberry (Sambucus nigra)
Black elderberry berries are used in treating colds and flu, and the flowers are known for their anti-inflammatory and cough-relieving effects.

Black Elderberry Syrup

Black elderberry syrup is commonly used to alleviate the symptoms of colds and flu.

Ingredients:
- 2 cups of ripe black elderberries
- 1 cup of water
- 1 cup of honey

Preparation: Place the berries and water in a pot and simmer on low heat for about 15-20 minutes. Strain the mixture to remove the berries, retaining the liquid. Mix the liquid with the honey, then heat on low for about 10 minutes. Store the finished syrup in a clean jar in the refrigerator.

Black Elderflower Infusion

Black elderflower infusion is known for its cough-relieving and antibacterial properties.

Ingredients:
- 2 tablespoons of dried black elderflowers
- 1 cup of boiling water

Preparation: Place the dried flowers in a teapot or cup. Pour boiling water over the flowers and leave to infuse for about 10 minutes. Strain the infusion and drink warm.

Vitamins: Black elder is particularly rich in vitamin C, which is a key component of immunity. It also contains B vitamins, including B6 and folates, which help in the proper functioning of the nervous system and the production of red blood cells.

Minerals: Elder is a source of potassium, which helps regulate blood pressure, and iron, which is essential for the production of hemoglobin. Antioxidants: Black elderberries are rich in antioxidants, including flavonoids and anthocyanins, which help protect the body from damage caused by free radicals.

Fiber: The fiber in black elderberries helps support the health of the digestive system, improves digestion, and regulates blood sugar levels.

Bioactive Compounds: Black elder also contains bioactive compounds such as phenolic acids and terpenes, which have a range of health benefits, including anti-inflammatory, antibacterial, and antiviral actions.

Remember that raw black elder can be toxic, so always properly process it before consumption. Although black elder has many health benefits, some parts of the plant, including unripe berries, can be toxic. Always properly process black elderberries before consumption.

Black elder, Sambucus nigra, was an important plant in the traditional medicine of the Vikings and ancient Europe. Its roots, leaves, flowers, and fruits were valued for a wide range of medicinal uses. The Vikings used elder flowers to produce medicinal drinks that helped combat symptoms of colds, flu, and other upper respiratory infections.

The fruit of the black elder, rich in antioxidants, was used to prepare juices, wines, and jams, which were utilized in the treatment of stomach ailments and as a general tonic. In ancient Europe, black elder was considered a magical plant whose presence brought protection and health, and its ability to support the immune system was valued as a gift from nature.

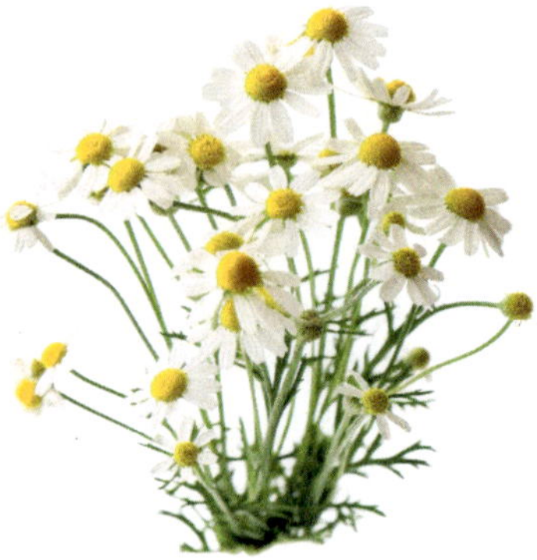

Chamomile (Matricaria chamomilla)
Chamomile is known for its calming and soothing properties, it helps with digestive problems and alleviates skin ailments. Chamomile is one of the most versatile herbs used in natural medicine. Its mild but effective action makes it suitable for people of all ages

<u>Chamomile Infusion</u>

A chamomile infusion is a classic way to utilize this herb. It helps to soothe digestive issues, reduces stress, and aids in sleep.

Ingredients:
- 1 teaspoon of dried chamomile
- 1 cup of boiling water

Preparation: Place the dried chamomile in a jug or cup. Pour boiling water over the chamomile and leave it to infuse for about 10 minutes. Strain the infusion and drink it warm.

Chamomile Oil

Chamomile oil can be applied topically to alleviate skin ailments such as irritations, rashes, or sunburn..

Ingredients:
- 1 cup of dried chamomile
- 2 cups of coconut oil or olive oil

Preparation: Place the dried chamomile in a jar, then pour the oil over it. Close the jar and leave it in a dark and cool place for 4-6 weeks, shaking daily. After this time, strain the oil into a clean jar. Store in a dark place. Apply to the skin as needed

Chamomile Bath

The calming properties of chamomile make it perfect for bathing. Adding a few drops of chamomile oil to warm bath water can help relax the mind and body, as well as alleviate skin ailments.

Hair Rinse

Chamomile is known for its ability to brighten and invigorate blonde hair. You can prepare a chamomile hair rinse by adding two tablespoons of dried flowers to one liter of water, boiling for 15 minutes, then straining. Rinse your hair with it after shampooing.

Chamomile Eye Compress

If you have puffy or tired eyes, a chamomile infusion can provide relief. Prepare a strong chamomile infusion (double the amount of dried chamomile per cup of boiling water), strain and let it cool. Soak cotton pads in the infusion and place them on closed eyelids for about 10 minutes.

Culinary Spice

Chamomile can also be added to various dishes. Dried flowers can be added to herbal tea, salads, sauces, or desserts, giving them a delicate, bittersweet taste.

Flavonoids: Chamomile contains numerous flavonoids, such as apigenin, quercetin, and luteolin, which have anti-inflammatory and anticancer properties. Terpenoids: Chamomile contains terpenoids, including bisabolol and chamazulene, which have strong anti-inflammatory and antibacterial properties.

Coumarins: Coumarins, such as herniarin and umbelliferone, have antispasmodic properties, which can help in the treatment of digestive disorders.

Polysaccharides: Polysaccharides present in chamomile can modulate the immune system, which can help in treating inflammatory conditions and allergies.

Vitamins and minerals: Chamomile also contains some amounts of vitamins, including vitamin C and some from the B group, as well as minerals such as potassium, calcium, magnesium, iron, and zinc. It is worth noting that chamomile is usually used in small amounts, so it is not a major source of vitamins and minerals in the diet. Its main health benefits come from the bioactive compounds it contains, which have strong anti-inflammatory, antibacterial, and calming properties.

Chamomile is a relatively strong herb and can dominate the taste of a dish, so use it sparingly..

Chamomile, also known as Matricaria chamomilla, was a key element in the herbal repertoire of Vikings and ancient Europe. This plant, recognizable by its bright, radiant inflorescences, was generously used in natural remedies.

The Vikings held chamomile in high regard, using it to alleviate various ailments, from digestive problems to insomnia.

A soft, soothing chamomile infusion, prepared by ancient warriors, helped to calm the mind after battle, and its anti-inflammatory properties were invaluable in wound treatment.

Interestingly, in many European cultures, chamomile was associated with the sun and was considered a symbol of renewal and regeneration, further confirming its ability to revitalize and rejuvenate the body and spirit.

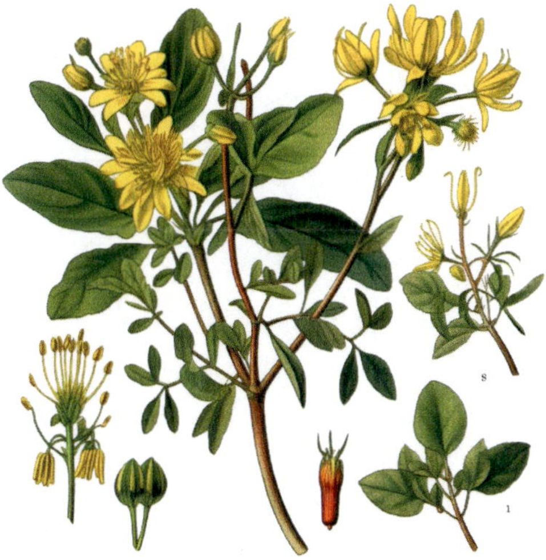

St. John's wort (Hypericum perforatum)
St. John's wort is often used to alleviate symptoms of depression and anxiety, as well as aiding in wound healing.

St. John's wort infusion

Ingredients:
- 2 teaspoons of dried St. John's wort
- 1 cup of boiling water

Preparation: Pour boiling water over the dried St. John's wort and leave for about 10 minutes to infuse. Strain the infusion. Done!

St. John's wort oil

Ingredients:
- Fresh St. John's wort flowers
- Olive oil

Preparation: Gather St. John's wort flowers, then place them in a jar, loosely, without pressing down. Pour olive oil over the flowers so that they are completely covered. Cover the jar and place it in a warm, sunny spot for about 6 weeks. After 6 weeks, strain the oil through a fine sieve or cloth. Store the prepared oil in a cool place, away from sunlight. You can drink St. John's wort infusion 1-2 times a day, and the oil can be applied externally to the skin for treating minor wounds, abrasions, or bruises.

St. John's wort tincture

It's easy to prepare and store.

Ingredients:
- Fresh or dried St. John's wort
- Vodka or spirits

Preparation: Put St. John's wort into a jar, filling it up to 3/4. Pour alcohol over the herb to the top, making sure the entire herb is submerged. Screw on the jar lid and place it in a dark, cool place for about 4-6 weeks. Shake the jar every few days. After this time, strain the tincture through a fine sieve or cloth into another jar or bottle. Store the tincture in a cool, dark place. St. John's wort tincture can be used internally to alleviate symptoms of anxiety and depression - always according to the recommendations of a specialist, as St. John's wort may interact with other medications. It can also be applied externally to the skin for treating minor wounds and burns.

Flavonoids: These are potent antioxidants that may help protect the body from free radicals and chronic diseases.

Hypericin and hyperoside: These chemical compounds are responsible for the antidepressant and anti-inflammatory properties of St. John's wort.

Tannins: These chemical compounds are responsible for the antidepressant and anti-inflammatory properties of St. John's wort.

Saponins: They have anti-inflammatory properties and may help protect the skin. Phytosterols: These are cholesterol-like compounds that may help lower LDL (low-density lipoprotein, „bad" cholesterol) levels in the blood.

Minerals: St. John's wort contains various minerals, such as potassium, calcium, magnesium, phosphorus, iron, and zinc.

However, remember that St. John's wort can interact with some medications, especially those such as antidepressants, anticoagulants, and hormonal drugs. If you are undergoing treatment, consult your doctor.

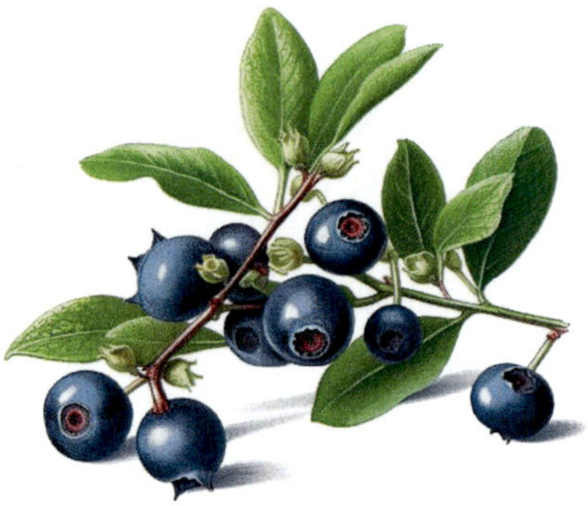

Bilberry (Vaccinium myrtillus)
Bilberries are rich in antioxidants that help protect the body from the harmful effects of free radicals. They also have antibacterial and anti--inflammatory properties.

Bilberry Juice

Bilberry juice is a delicious and healthy way to consume these fruits.

Ingredients:
- 2 cups of fresh black bilberries
- 1/4 cup of water
- 1-2 tablespoons of honey (optional)

Preparation: Wash the bilberries and put them in a pot. Add water and simmer over low heat for about 10 minutes, until the bilberries begin to burst and release juice. Strain through a fine mesh sieve to remove skins and seeds. Season with honey to taste, if desired. Pour the juice into a bottle and store in the refrigerator. The juice is best fresh, but it can be stored in the refrigerator for a few days.

Bilberry Jam

Bilberry jam is a classic recipe that lets you enjoy the taste of bilberries all year round.

Ingredients:
- 4 cups of fresh bilberries
- 1 cup of sugar
- Juice from 1/2 lemon

Preparation: Wash the bilberries and place them in a large pot. Add sugar and lemon juice, stir. Cook over medium heat, stirring occasionally, until the jam starts to thicken. When the jam reaches the desired consistency, pour it into sterilized jars. Close the jars and turn them upside down to create a vacuum seal. After cooling, store in a cool, dark place.

Fresh Bilberries with Yogurt and Honey

A simple and healthy dessert that can be prepared in a few minutes.

Ingredients:
- 1 cup of fresh bilberries
- 1 cup of natural yogurt
- 1-2 tablespoons of honey

Preparation: Wash the bilberries and place them in a bowl. Add yogurt and honey to taste. Stir and enjoy a healthy, straightforwardly prepared dessert.

Vitamins: Bilberries are a rich source of vitamins, especially vitamin C, which is a potent antioxidant. They also contain vitamin A, and B group vitamins such as B1 (thiamine), B2 (riboflavin), B3 (niacin), B6, and vitamin K.

Minerals: Bilberries contain many minerals, including manganese, which is crucial for bone health and aids in the metabolism of sugars and fats. They also contain potassium, copper, iron, zinc, and magnesium.

Antioxidants: Bilberries are rich in antioxidants, particularly anthocyanins, which give them their distinctive dark color. Anthocyanins help combat free radicals in the body, which can contribute to reducing the risk of many chronic diseases, such as heart disease and cancer.

Fiber: Bilberries are also an excellent source of fiber, which helps in regulating digestion and can contribute to maintaining a healthy body weight.

Plant Compounds: Bilberries also contain other important plant compounds, such as ellagic acid, quercetin, and resveratrol, which may contribute to improving heart, brain, and digestive health.

Overall, bilberries are one of the healthiest fruits you can consume, and their regular consumption can contribute to improving overall health and well-being.

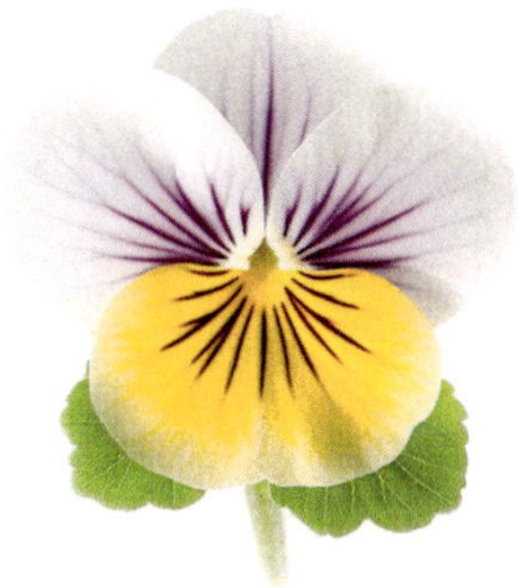

Field/Tricolor Violet (Viola arvensis and Viola tricolor)
Used for treating skin conditions, but also as a calming and antibacterial agent.

Violet Flower Infusion

Ingredients:
- 2 teaspoons of dried violet flowers
- 1 cup of boiling water

Preparation: Add the dried flowers to a cup of boiling water. Allow the infusion to steep for about 10 minutes. Strain the infusion and it's ready to drink.

Violet Skin Rinse

Ingredients:
- 1/2 cup of dried violet flowers
- 1 liter of boiling water

Preparation: Add dried flowers to a liter of boiling water. Allow the infusion to cool down. Strain the infusion, it's ready to use as a face rinse or bath additive.

Violet Salve

Ingredients:
- 1 cup of fresh violet flowers
- 1 cup of coconut oil
- 1/4 cup of beeswax

Preparation: Add fresh flowers to a cup of coconut oil. Heat on low for about 3 hours. Strain the oil, remove the flowers. Add beeswax to the oil, heat on low until you get a uniform mass. Allow the salve to cool down, it is now ready to use.

Flavonoids: These are powerful antioxidants that can protect the body from the harmful effects of free radicals. Flavonoids may support heart and brain health and may have anti-cancer properties.

Tannins: They have anti-inflammatory and antibacterial effects. They may help in the treatment of inflammatory conditions of the skin and mucous membranes.

Saponins: These are chemical compounds with antifungal and antibacterial effects. They can assist in the treatment of various infections.

Salicylic Acid: This is a natural anti-inflammatory ingredient that can help in the treatment of inflammatory skin conditions, such as acne and eczema.

Fumaric Acid: This is a compound that is often used in the treatment of psoriasis.

Vitamin C: This is a potent antioxidant that supports the immune system, collagen production, and skin health.

Carotenoids: These are plant pigments that can act as antioxidants. They can support eye, skin, and immune system health..

Remember that when preparing an infusion or extract from tricolor violet, some of these ingredients may break down under high temperature. Therefore, it's always important to be careful and understand well what benefits can be obtained from a given compound and how to make the best use of it.

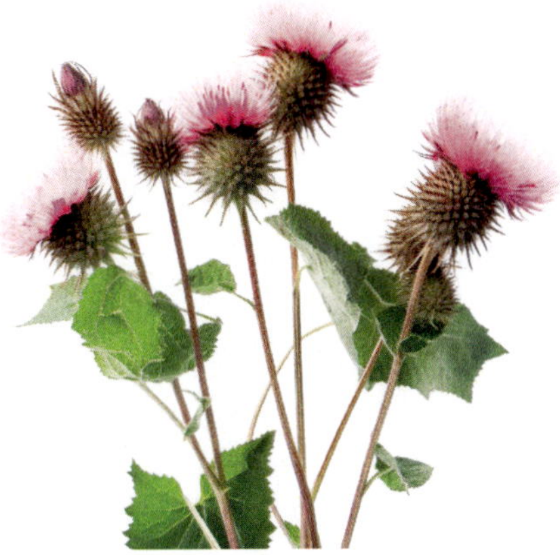

Great Burdock (Arctium lappa)
Burdock is known as a detoxifying agent, accelerating wound healing and soothing skin problems.

Decoction of burdock root

Ingredients:
- 2 tablespoons of dried burdock root
- 1 liter of water

Preparation: Place the dried burdock root in a pot. Add water and bring to a boil. Reduce the heat to a minimum and simmer for about 15 minutes. After cooking, strain the decoction to remove the root. The decoction can be consumed hot or cold. Store it in the refrigerator for a maximum of 3 days. Burdock root decoction is particularly effective in detoxifying the body.

It contains inulin, a natural prebiotic, which supports healthy gut flora and aids in removing toxins from the body. Thanks to its anti-inflammatory properties, burdock root decoction can also accelerate wound healing and soothe skin inflammations. It can be used as a natural aid in the treatment of acne, eczema, psoriasis, and other skin problems.

Burdock oil

Ingredients:
- Fresh burdock root
- Base oil (e.g., olive oil, coconut oil)

Preparation: Wash the burdock root and cut it into thin slices. Place the root slices in a jar and pour in the base oil, so they are completely covered. Tightly close the jar and set it aside in a warm, dark place for about 4-6 weeks. After this time, strain the oil to remove the root. Store the ready oil in a dark bottle in a cool place. It can be applied externally to the skin. Before using the oil on the skin, conduct an allergy test by applying a small amount to the skin and observing the reaction for 24 hours. If any signs of irritation or allergy appear, do not use the oil.

Burdock oil is valued for its abilities to soothe skin inflammations. It is rich in a fatty acid called arachidonic acid, which is a known antioxidant. When applied to the skin, burdock oil can counteract dryness, itching, and redness of the skin. Its regular use can help reduce the symptoms of psoriasis, eczema, and other inflammatory skin conditions. In addition, burdock oil is often used in hair care, as it can stimulate hair growth and reduce hair loss.

Inulin: This natural substance is present in burdock in large amounts, especially in the root. Inulin is a prebiotic that supports healthy gut flora and aids in the detoxification of the body.

Polyphenols: Burdock contains various polyphenols, which have strong antioxidant and anti-inflammatory properties.

Minerals: Burdock is a good source of many minerals, such as potassium, magnesium, calcium, and iron.

Vitamins: Burdock also contains vitamins, especially B-group vitamins and vitamin C.

Fatty acids: Burdock oil is rich in unsaturated fatty acids, including linoleic acid and oleic acid, which are beneficial for the health of the skin and hair.

Arachidonic acid: This is a type of unsaturated fatty acid that has strong anti-inflammatory properties.

Remember, the nutritional components in burdock can vary depending on the growing conditions and processing of the plant. To enjoy the full range of health benefits of burdock, always look for high-quality products.

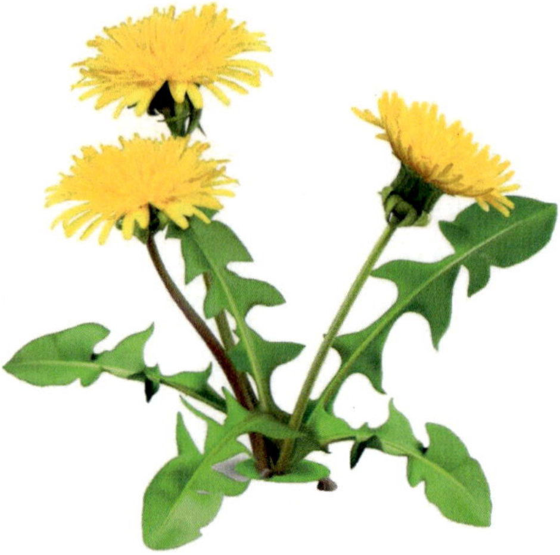

Dandelion (Taraxacum officinale)
Dandelion is used as a diuretic, as well as for detoxifying the body and aiding digestion.

Dandelion Leaf Infusion

Ingredients:
- 1 tablespoon of dried dandelion leaves
- 1 cup of water

Preparation: Boil a cup of water. Add a tablespoon of dried dandelion leaves to the hot water. Cover and leave to steep for about 10 minutes. Strain the infusion and serve warm. Dandelion is also popularly used in salad form. Young leaves can be harvested in the spring and added to salads for extra flavor and health benefits.

Dandelion Salad

Ingredients:
- 2 cups of young dandelion leaves
- 1 cup of other salad leaves (e.g., arugula, spinach)
- 1 tomato
- 1 cucumber
- 1/4 onion
- salad dressing of choice (e.g., olive oil, balsamic vinegar)

Preparation: Wash the dandelion leaves and other salad leaves thoroughly. Cut the tomato, cucumber, and onion into pieces. Mix all the ingredients together and drizzle with salad dressing. Always remember to gather dandelion from clean areas, away from pollution and pesticides.

Dandelion Tincture

Ingredients:
2 cups of fresh dandelion flowers
1 liter of vodka or spirits
A jar with a capacity of 1.5 liters
Dark, glass bottles for storage

Preparation: Carefully wash and dry the dandelion flowers. Place the flowers in the jar, then pour over the vodka or spirits. Close the jar and set aside in a dark, cool place for about 4 weeks.

After this time, strain the tincture through a cheesecloth into a dark glass bottle, trying to separate the liquid from the flowers as thoroughly as possible. Store in a dark place.

Dandelion tincture can be consumed in small amounts, such as one teaspoon before a meal, to aid digestion. However, remember that despite their medicinal properties, herbal tinctures are also strong alcohol and should be consumed in moderation.

Vitamins: It is an excellent source of vitamins A, C, D, and K. Vitamin A is known for its benefits to eye health, while vitamin C is a strong antioxidant that supports the immune system. Vitamin D is necessary for bone and teeth health, and vitamin K aids blood clotting.

Minerals: Dandelion is rich in minerals such as potassium, iron, calcium, and magnesium. Potassium regulates blood pressure and the body's water balance, iron is essential for the production of hemoglobin, calcium is key for bone and teeth health, and magnesium supports nerve and muscle functions.

Fiber: Dandelion contains inulin, a type of prebiotic fiber, which is beneficial for gut health. Inulin supports the growth of beneficial gut microflora, which positively affects the health of the entire body.

Flavonoids: Dandelion also contains flavonoids, which are potent antioxidants. Flavonoids help protect the body from harmful free radicals.

Phenolic acid and coumarins: These compounds have strong antioxidant and anti-inflammatory properties, which help protect the body against various diseases.

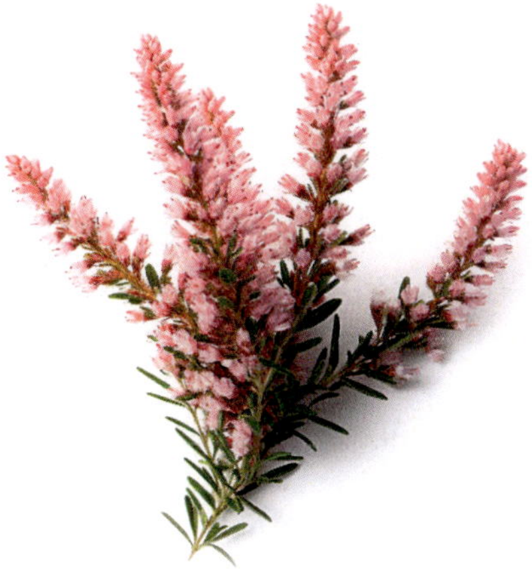

Common Heather (Calluna vulgaris)
Heather is used to treat urinary and kidney infections, as well as a pain reliever.

Heather Infusion

Ingredients:
- 1 tablespoon of dried heather flowers
- 1 cup of boiling water

Preparation: Put the dried flowers into a mug. Pour over with boiling water and cover, then leave to brew for about 10 minutes. Strain the infusion and let it cool down. You can drink 2-3 cups of this infusion daily, especially if you suffer from urinary system problems.

Heather Tincture

Ingredients:
- 1 cup of dried heather flowers
- 500 of spirit (40% alcohol)

Preparation: Place the flowers in a jar. Pour the spirit over the flowers until they are fully covered. Screw on the lid and leave it in a dark, cool place for 2-3 weeks. After this time, strain the tincture and store it in a dark place. The tincture can be applied externally to painful spots or internally - 1 teaspoon 2-3 times
a day.

Treating urinary tract infections: Heather has diuretic effects, which means it helps the body produce more urine. This is particularly beneficial for people suffering from urinary tract infections, such as cystitis, as it may assist in flushing bacteria out of the urinary system. Supporting kidney disease treatment: It also acts as a diuretic, assisting in the removal of excess fluids from the body. This can be beneficial for people with kidney issues, such as kidney stones.

Pain relief: Heather has analgesic properties, meaning it can help relieve pain. This can be especially helpful for people suffering from chronic diseases, such as rheumatoid arthritis.

Anti-inflammatory: Heather also has anti-inflammatory properties, which can help alleviate inflammatory conditions in the body, such as arthritis. Support for cardiovascular health: Heather is also used to support cardiovascular health, assisting in blood pressure regulation and improving overall heart function.

Flavonoids: Heather contains flavonoids, which are powerful antioxidants and have anti-inflammatory effects. They may help protect the body from damage caused by free radicals and chronic inflammatory conditions

Triterpenes: Heather also contains triterpenes, which have a range of potential health benefits, including anticancer, antiviral, antibacterial, and anti-inflammatory effects

Arbutin: Heather is one of the few sources of arbutin - a compound that has strong diuretic and antiseptic properties.

Phenolic acids: Heather also contains phenolic acids, which have strong antioxidant and anticancer effects.

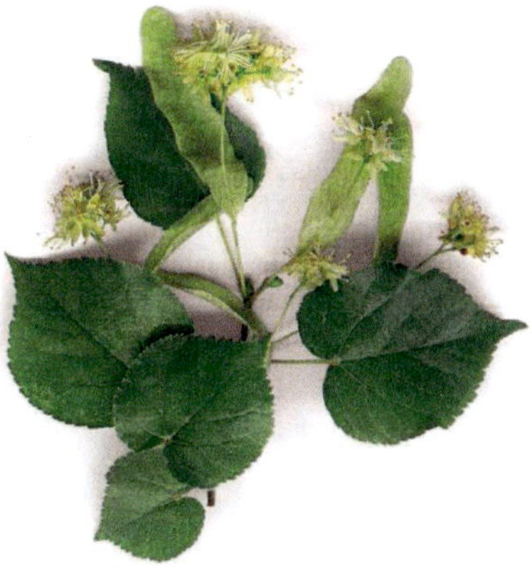

Small-leaved Lime (Tilia cordata)

Linden is known for its calming properties and support in sleep. It is also used to alleviate respiratory tract infections.

Linden Flower Infusion

Ingredients:

- 2 tablespoons of dried linden flowers
- 1 cup of water

Preparation: Boil the water and pour it over the linden flowers in a te-apot or mug. Leave to steep for about 10 minutes. Strain and drink 1-2 times a day. Linden flower infusion helps combat stress and tension, and also aids in sleep issues. .

Linden Flower Juice

Ingredients:
- 4 cups of fresh linden flowers
- 1 liter of water
- 1 kilogram of sugar or 8 large tablespoons of honey

Preparation: Transfer linden flowers to a large pot, cover with water, and simmer on low heat for about 15 minutes. Add sugar and continue to cook for about 15 minutes, until the sugar has completely dissolved. Strain the finished juice through a sieve, then pour into clean bottles. Store in a cool place. Linden flower juice can be added to tea or drunk solo to alleviate cough and cold symptoms.

Linden Flower Tincture

Ingredients:
- 1 cup of fresh linden flowers
- 500 ml of spirit (40% alcohol)
- 250 ml of water
- 200 g of sugar or honey

Preparation: Wash and dry the linden flowers, then transfer them to a jar. Pour the flowers with the spirit and close the jar. Leave it in a dark place for 2 weeks, shaking the jar daily. After this time, prepare a sugar syrup. Add water and sugar to a pot, cook on low heat until the sugar dissolves. Let it cool down. Strain the spirit from the flowers into a separate vessel, then combine it with the sugar syrup. Mix. Pour the tincture into bottles and store in a dark place. Linden flower tincture has calming, antiviral and anti-inflammatory effects.

It can be used to alleviate the symptoms of cold and flu, as well as to calm down and improve sleep. However, due to the alcohol content, it should be consumed in moderation. Herbal tinctures, although natural, can be stronger than infusions.

Sleep problems and insomnia: Linden flowers have a calming effect, which aids in relaxation and facilitates falling asleep. This can be particularly helpful for people suffering from insomnia or stress.

Upper respiratory tract infections: Linden flowers have antibacterial and anti-inflammatory effects that can help in treating upper respiratory tract infections such as cold and flu.

Hypertension: Linden flowers can help lower blood pressure, which is beneficial for people suffering from hypertension.

Inflammation and pain: An infusion of linden flowers has analgesic properties that can help alleviate inflammation and pain.

Digestive problems: Linden flowers can help improve digestion and reduce symptoms such as bloating, heartburn, and indigestion.

Flavonoids: Linden flowers contain a large amount of flavonoids, which are known antioxidants. Antioxidants help fight free radicals, which can cause cell damage and contribute to the development of many diseases, including heart diseases and cancers.

Phenolic Acid: This substance has strong anti-inflammatory and antioxidant properties.

Tiliacin: Tiliacin is a compound that has calming and anti-anxiety effects..

Plant Mucilages: Linden flowers contain mucilages that can soothe irritations of the mucous membranes, which is especially beneficial in the case of respiratory tract infections..

Eucalyptol: This ingredient, also known as 1,8-cineol, aids in the treatment of respiratory system infections, thanks to its anti-inflammatory, antibacterial and expectorant properties

Vitamins and minerals: Linden flowers also contain various vitamins and minerals, including vitamin C and potassium.

The linden flower, with its delicate but intense fragrance, was valued by European peoples, including the Vikings, for its wealth in compounds with medicinal properties. Traditionally used as a calming, antipyretic and diaphoretic agent, the linden flower remains an integral part of natural medicine, allowing us to reap the same benefits as our ancestors..

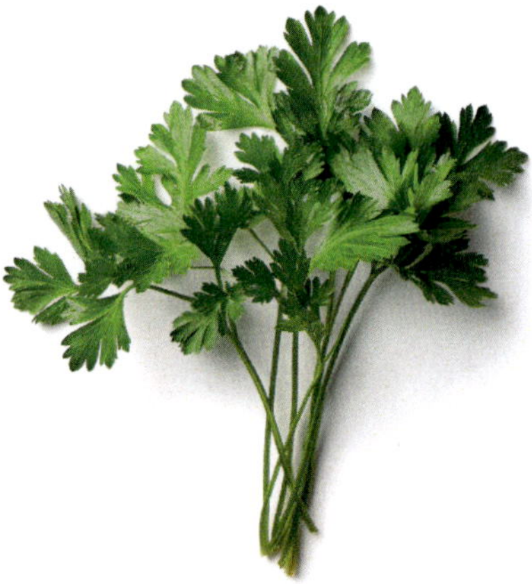

Common Parsley (Petroselinum crispum)
Parsley was used as a diuretic to support kidney function and cleanse the body. Parsley is extremely versatile, not only as an addition to various dishes, but also as a component of natural remedies.

Parsley Infusion

Ingredients:

- 2 tablespoons of freshly chopped parsley
- 250 ml of boiling water

Preparation: Add chopped parsley to a teapot. Pour boiling water over it and let it steep for about 10 minutes. Strain the infusion and drink it. You can add a little honey for improved taste. Parsley infusion is beneficial for the urinary system and helps to cleanse the body.

Green Parsley Smoothie

Ingredients:
- 1 bunch of fresh parsley
- 1 apple
- 1 cucumber
- Juice from half a lemon
- 250 ml of water

Preparation: Wash all ingredients, chop the apple and cucumber into smaller pieces. Put everything into the blender and blend until smooth. The smoothie is ready to consume. Such a smoothie is rich in vitamins and minerals, and parsley adds cleansing properties to it.

Parsley Honey

Ingredients:
- 1 bunch of fresh parsley
- 1 cup of honey

Preparation: Finely chop the parsley and place it in a jar. Pour in honey so as to completely cover the parsley. Mix and close the jar. Store in a dark, cool place for two weeks, stirring the contents of the jar daily.

After two weeks, strain and store the obtained parsley honey in the refrigerator. Such honey can be used for sore throat or urinary tract infections.

Parsley as an addition to salads

You can simply add it to salads to enhance the flavor and as a source of additional vitamins and minerals.

Parsley can also be added to post-workout protein shakes

Parsley is rich in vitamin C, which aids in the absorption of iron, and it is also a source of magnesium, which is essential for healthy muscles.

Parsley Poultice

Parsley is used in cosmetics to alleviate swelling and bruises. We can make a simple parsley poultice to apply to the skin.

Ingredients:
- 1 bunch of fresh parsley
- 1 tablespoon of olive oil

Preparation: Finely chop the parsley and place it in the mask. Add olive oil and mix until you get a paste consistency. Apply the poultice to the skin for 10-15 minutes, then rinse with warm water.

Parsley Tincture

Ingredients:
- 1 bunch of fresh parsley
- 500 ml of vodka

Preparation: Finely chop the parsley and place it in a jar. Pour in vodka so that it completely covers the parsley. Close the jar and store in a dark, cool place for two weeks. After this time, strain the tincture. Parsley tincture can be used externally for bruises and also orally as a digestive aid and for detoxifying the body.

Detox Green Smoothie with Parsley

This smoothie is full of vitamins and nutrients that will help cleanse your body and boost your energy.

Ingredients:
- 1 bunch of fresh parsley
- 1 apple
- 1 cucumber
- 1 lemon
- A piece of fresh ginger
- 1 cup of water

Preparation: Thoroughly wash all ingredients, peel and cut into smaller pieces. Put everything in a blender and blend until you reach a uniform consistency. If the smoothie is too thick, add more water. The finished smoothie is best consumed immediately after preparation.

Parsley Tea with Honey and Lemon

Parsley tea has many health benefits, such as aiding digestion and cleansing the body.

Ingredients:
- 2 tablespoons of fresh parsley
- Juice of 1/2 lemon
- 1 teaspoon of honey
- 250 ml of water

Preparation: Boil water in a kettle or pot. Finely chop the parsley and place it in a cup. Pour over hot water and let it brew for about 10 minutes. After this time, add lemon juice and honey. Parsley tea is ready to drink. You can drink it 1-2 times a day.

Vitamin K: Parsley is one of the best sources of this vitamin, which is crucial for bone health and blood clotting.

Vitamin C: This is a powerful antioxidant that supports the immune system, as well as skin health.

Vitamin A: The beta-carotene found in parsley is converted into vitamin A in the body, which helps maintain healthy eyes and skin.

Folate (Vitamin B9): This is a key nutrient that helps in the production and repair of DNA, as well as in the production of red blood cells.

Iron: Parsley is a good source of iron, which helps in the production of hemoglobin, a component of red blood cells.

Calcium: This mineral is essential for healthy bones and teeth

Potassium: This mineral helps control blood pressure and ensures the heart functions properly.

In the emerald thicket of parsley leaves lies the secret to health, which European peoples discovered many centuries ago in natural medicine.

Going beyond the role of a decorative addition to dishes, parsley was considered a powerful element in the natural medicine cabinet, providing not only an intense taste, but also various health benefits.

The wealth of vitamins and minerals, including the extremely valuable vitamin C and iron, made parsley an important part of the diet, supporting the immune system and improving the functioning of the body. Used both fresh and dried, parsley deserves a place in every kitchen and medicine cabinet, allowing us to connect with the traditions of our ancestors and benefit from the gifts of nature in caring for our health.

Regardless of whether you add it to soup or prepare a mixture based on it, parsley reminds us that nature provides us with everything we need to live healthily and in harmony with the rhythm of nature.

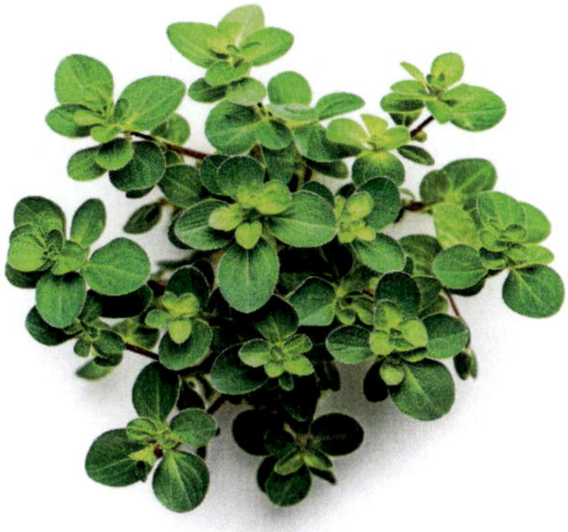

Sweet Marjoram (Origanum majorana)
Marjoram has strong antibacterial, antiviral, and antifungal properties. It finds its use in both medicine and cooking.

Marjoram Infusion

Ingredients:
- 2 teaspoons of dried marjoram
- 1 cup of boiling water

Preparation: Add two teaspoons of dried marjoram to a cup of boiling water. Cover and leave to steep for about 10 minutes. Strain the infusion and drink it. A marjoram infusion can help alleviate gastrointestinal ailments such as bloating, stomach pain, or indigestion.

Marjoram oil:

You can prepare marjoram oil at home using a process of maceration, which involves immersing marjoram in oil to extract its active ingredients.

Ingredients:

- 1 cup of dried marjoram
- 2 cups of extra virgin olive oil (or any other oil with a neutral taste, such as coconut oil or sunflower oil)

Preparation: Place the dried marjoram in a jar. Pour the oil over the marjoram, ensuring that all the leaves are completely submerged. Cover the jar and place it in a warm, dark place for about 2-3 weeks. You can shake the jar every few days to ensure even extraction of the ingredients from the marjoram. After 2-3 weeks, strain the oil through a fine sieve or cheesecloth into a clean jar, separating the marjoram leaves. The oil should have a strong marjoram aroma. Store the oil in a dark, cool place. Use it as needed, for example, on the skin or as an addition to dishes.

Marjoram oil is used as a natural remedy for muscle and joint pain. It can be added to baths or used as a massage ingredient. Its strong antibacterial and antiviral properties make it effective in treating skin and respiratory infections.

Food Additive: Marjoram is also commonly used as a spice in cooking. It is added to sauces, soups, meats, and other dishes, which not only enriches their flavor but also provides beneficial nutrients.

Vitamins: Marjoram is a good source of vitamins such as vitamin C, vitamin A, vitamin K, and some of the B vitamins, including niacin, pyridoxine (B6), and folates.

Minerals: This aromatic herbal addition to dishes is also a source of many important minerals, including calcium, iron, manganese, magnesium, potassium, and zinc.

Fiber: Marjoram contains fiber, which is beneficial for the health of the digestive system and can help prevent constipation.

Antioxidants: Marjoram also contains plant compounds with antioxidant properties, which may help combat free radicals in the body. These antioxidants include various flavonoids and phenolic compounds.

Thymol and Carvacrol: These two phytochemicals have strong antibacterial and antifungal properties, making marjoram a powerful tool in the fight against various pathogens

Rosmarinic Acid: This bioactive compound is known for its anticancer, anti-inflammatory, antidiabetic, and neuroprotective properties.

Terpenes: Marjoram contains many different terpenes, which are natural compounds found in plants, known for their strong anti-inflammatory and anticancer properties.

Estragole: A compound that may act as a natural antibacterial and antiviral agent.

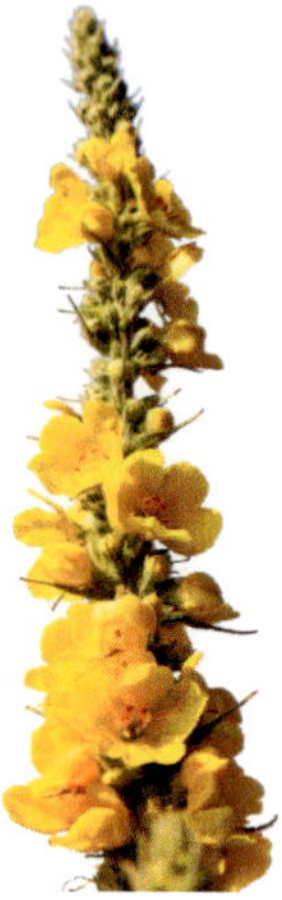

Mullein Flower (Verbascum)

Mullein flower was traditionally used to soothe coughs and other respiratory ailments. Mullein flower, also known as „the king of medicinal plants," has been used in natural medicine for centuries. There are records of its use by the ancient Greeks and Romans, suggesting it may have been in use for at least 2000 years.

Mullein Flower Syrup

Ingredients:

- 2 cups of fresh mullein flowers
- 1 cup of water
- 1 cup of honey

Preparation: Place the mullein flowers and water in a pot and simmer over low heat for about 15 minutes. Strain the mixture to remove the flowers, keeping the liquid. Add the honey to the liquid, then heat over low heat for about 10 minutes. Store the finished syrup in a clean jar in the refrigerator. Mullein flower syrup is traditionally used to soothe coughs and other respiratory ailments, such as asthma and bronchitis.

Mullein Flower Tincture

Ingredients:
- 1 cup of fresh mullein flowers
- 2 cups of strong vodka

Preparation: Place the mullein flowers in a jar, then pour over the vodka. Seal the jar and leave it in a dark, cool place for at least 2 weeks. After this time, strain the tincture, removing the flowers. Store the tincture in a clean bottle in a dark place.

Mullein flower tincture can be used externally to treat inflammatory skin conditions such as eczema. It may also provide relief for muscular and joint pains. Internally, the tincture can be used as a cough suppressant.

Mullein Flower Oil

Ingredients:
- 1 cup of fresh mullein flowers
- 2 cups of coconut oil (you can also use sweet almond oil or olive oil)

Preparation: Place the mullein flowers in a jar. Pour over your chosen oil to completely cover the flowers. Seal the jar and leave it in a dark, cool place for at least 2 weeks. After this time, strain the oil, removing the flowers. Store the oil in a clean bottle.

Mullein flower oil can be applied topically to the skin to soothe inflammatory conditions such as eczema, and to treat minor wounds and burns. The antibacterial and anti-inflammatory properties of mullein flowers make the oil effective for treating acne as well.

Iridoid glycosides - these are natural chemical compounds found in many different types of plants. They have anti-inflammatory, antibacterial, and antiviral effects.

Saponins - hese are compounds that have a mucolytic effect, which means they help to thin and remove mucus from the respiratory tract. That's why mullein is often used in treating coughs..

Flavonoids - these are compounds that have strong antioxidant properties. They help protect the body from the harmful effects of free radicals.

Mucilage - it is present in large amounts in mullein flowers. It is soothing for the mucous membranes, hence its use in alleviating coughs and other respiratory complaints.

Triterpenes: These compounds have anti-inflammatory and antibacterial effects.

Coumarins: These are organic compounds that may have antibacterial, antiviral, anti-inflammatory, and antioxidative effects.

Coumarins: These are organic compounds that can have antibacterial, antiviral, anti-inflammatory, and antioxidant effects.

Polyphenols: These are chemical compounds that have antioxidant action and may help protect the body from damage caused by free radicals.

Plant sterols: They may contribute to heart and circulatory health. Minerals: Mullein also contains small amounts of various minerals, such as copper, zinc, manganese, magnesium, potassium, phosphorus, and calcium.

Vitamins: Although mullein is not typically known as a rich source of vitamins, it contains small amounts of some, such as vitamins B1, B2, C, and E. Mullein, sensually spreading its bright yellow flowers under the summer sun, played a key role in the herbal medicine cabinet of the Vikings and ancient European communities. Its fleeting scent translated into powerful healing properties - endowed with calming power and the ability to soothe piercing joint pains.

It was a plant of wisdom beyond its beauty, whispering the secrets of nature-aligned health to those who were ready to listen

❖

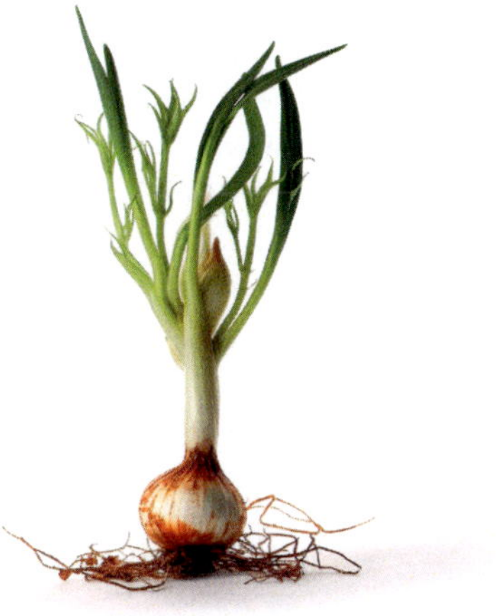

Onion (Allium cepa)
Onions have strong antibacterial and anti-inflammatory properties, they are also known for blood cleansing and improving heart function.

Onion Syrup

Onion has natural anti-inflammatory properties and can help alleviate cough.

Ingredients:
- 1 large onion
- 2-3 tablespoons of honey

Preparation: Chop the onion into small pieces and place it in a small saucepan. Keep in mind that the onion will release water, but you can add a minimal amount of water to avoid burning the sugar. Add honey to the onion and cook on low heat until the onion softens. Allow the syrup to cool, then strain it, discarding the onion. Store the syrup in the refrigerator and use it for cough relief, taking 1 tablespoon every 3-4 hours.

Onion syrup is a traditional home remedy for cough that has been used for a long time. Onions have anti-inflammatory properties and can help soothe throat irritation, which often accompanies a cough. Honey also has a soothing effect on the throat and possesses anti-inflammatory properties. Onion syrup can be particularly helpful for relieving dry cough, which provides no relief.

Onion juice for boosting immunity

Onions contain large amounts of vitamin C, which is necessary for maintaining a healthy immune system.

Ingredients:
- large onion
- 1 cup of water

Preparation: Chop the onion into small pieces and place in a blender. Add water and blend until you have a uniform consistency. Strain the juice through a fine sieve or cloth, discarding the onion remnants. You can drink onion juice on an empty stomach, up to 1 cup per day.

Onion juice contains a large amount of vitamin C, which is necessary for maintaining a healthy immune system. Regular consumption of onion juice may help increase immunity and protect against infections. However, it's worth noting that onion juice has a strong taste, which some people might not enjoy.

Onion Compress for Swelling and Bruises

Onion has natural anti-inflammatory properties and can help reduce swelling and pain associated with bruises.

Ingredients:

- 1 fresh onion

Preparation: Cut the onion into thin slices. Place the onion slices directly on the bruise or swelling. Secure in place with a bandage and leave on for about 2 hours.

Onion is known for its natural analgesic and anti-inflammatory properties. Onion compresses can help reduce swelling and pain associated with bruises and injuries. Onion may also help speed up the healing process.

Onion Tincture

Ingredients:

- 1 large onion
- 500 ml of spirits
- 250 g of sugar

Preparation: Peel and chop the onion into small pieces. Place the chopped onion in a glass jar. Add sugar and spirits. Close the jar and shake a few times to combine the ingredients. Store the jar in a dark place for about 2 weeks, stirring the contents daily. After 2 weeks, strain the tincture, discarding the onion. Store the tincture in a dark bottle.

Onion tincture can be used as a remedy to alleviate the symptoms of colds, flu, and also support digestion. *Due to the alcohol content, it should be used moderately.* Onion tincture is used as a home remedy for various ailments, such as colds, flu, or digestive problems.

Vitamins: Vitamin C: This powerful antioxidant vitamin supports the immune system, speeds up wound healing, and helps in the production of collagen, which is key for skin health.

B Vitamins: Onion is a good source of B vitamins B1 (thiamine), B2 (riboflavin), B3 (niacin), B5 (pantothenic acid), B6 (pyridoxine), and B9 (folates), which are essential for proper metabolism, energy production, and nervous system health.

Vitamin A: This vitamin is crucial for eye health, skin health, and immune system health.

Minerals - **Potassiums**: This mineral is necessary for the proper functioning of muscles, including the heart muscle, and regulating blood pressure..
Sulfur: Sulfur in onions has detoxifying properties and is key to the production of glutathione, one of the most important antioxidants in our body..
Phosphorus, calcium, and magnesium: These minerals are essential for bone and tooth health, and magnesium additionally supports the proper functioning of muscles and the nervous system.

Iron: Is necessary for the production of hemoglobin, the protein that carries oxygen in red blood cells.

Quercetin: This is a powerful antioxidant that can act as an anti-inflammatory, antihistamine, and lower blood pressure.

Sulfuric cysteine: This substance helps in the detoxification of the body, especially from heavy metals.

Fructans: These prebiotics support healthy gut bacteria.

Fiber: Supports digestion and helps regulate blood sugar levels.

Onion, an incredibly popular vegetable in our kitchen, has long been valued by Vikings and other peoples of Europe for its strong medicinal properties. Rich in antioxidants and sulfur compounds, onion has powerful antibacterial properties, making it often used to treat infections and speed up wound healing. The Vikings also appreciated the onion as an effective painkiller and antipyretic, reminding us of the invaluable value of this common vegetable in natural medicine.

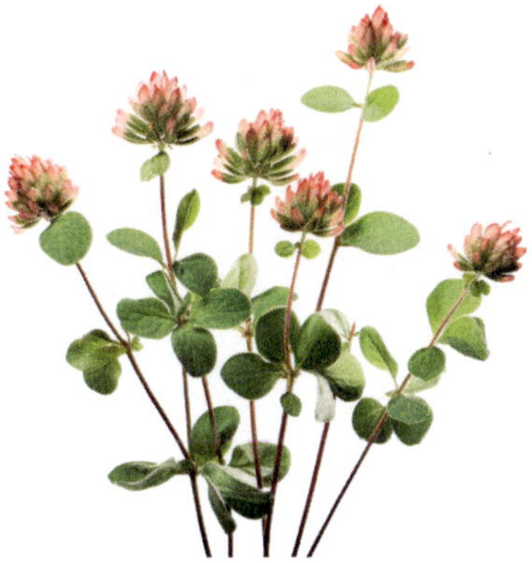

Red Clover (Trifolium pratense)
Red clover is used in the treatment of inflammatory skin conditions, but also as a remedy to alleviate menopause symptoms.

<u>Red Clover Infusion</u>

Ingredients:
- 1-2 tablespoons of dried red clover flowers
- 1 cup of boiling water

Preparation: Place the dried flowers in a cup. Pour over boiling water and cover. Let it steep for 10-15 minutes. Strain before consumption.

An infusion of red clover is known for its properties that alleviate menopausal symptoms, such as hot flashes, night sweats, and mood disorders. Moreover, red clover is rich in isoflavones - plant compounds that mimic the action of estrogen in the body. Therefore, a red clover infusion can also be helpful in treating other hormone-related conditions, such as PMS or irregular menstrual cycles.

Red Clover Tincture

Ingredients:
- 1 dried red clover flowers
- 500 ml of spirits (40% alcohol)

Preparation: Place the clover flowers in a glass jar. Pour over the spirits, ensuring that the flowers are completely covered by the liquid. Close the jar and shake it several times. Leave in a dark place for about 4-6 weeks, shaking the jar daily. After this time, strain the liquid through a gauze into a clean jar.

The tincture can be applied externally for the treatment of inflammatory skin conditions such as eczema or psoriasis. When taken internally, it can help alleviate menopausal symptoms.

Remember, however, that red clover contains phytohormones, which can affect hormone levels in the body. For this reason, caution should be exercised when using it, especially in people with present or suspected hormone-dependent cancer, such as breast, ovarian, or prostate cancer.

Isoflavones: Red clover is one of the richest sources of isoflavones, plant compounds in the group of phytoestrogens. Isoflavones, such as biochanin A, formononetin, daidzein, and genistein, mimic the action of estrogen in the body, which can help alleviate menopausal symptoms.

Saponins: These plant compounds may have anti-inflammatory effects, making red clover helpful in treating various inflammatory conditions, including skin inflammations.

Polyphenols: Red clover also contains polyphenols, including flavonoids and phenolic acids, which have antioxidant, anti-inflammatory, and anticancer effects.

Vitamins and minerals: Red clover is a source of many vitamins and minerals, including vitamin C, B vitamins, folic acid, calcium, magnesium, potassium, iron, and zinc.

Protein: Red clover is also quite rich in protein, especially compared to other herbal plants

Coumestans: These are other phytoestrogens present in red clover that can influence hormonal balance in the body.

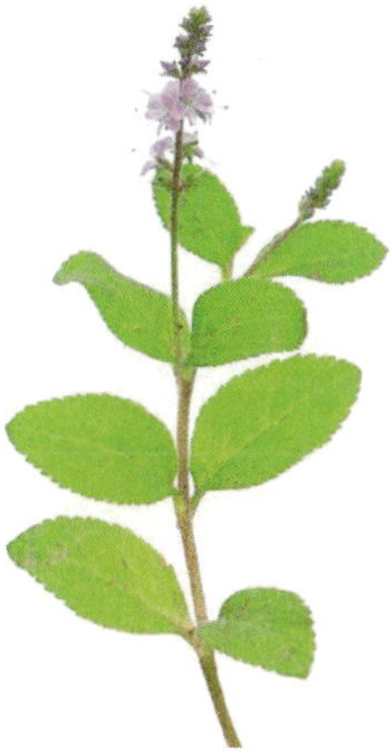

Heath Speedwell (Veronica officinalis))
Known for its antibacterial and anti-inflammatory properties, heath speedwell has been used to treat upper respiratory tract infections..

Heath Speedwell Tea

Ingredients:
- 1-2 teaspoons of dried heath speedwell
- 1 cup of boiling water

Preparation: Place the dried herb into a cup. Pour over the boiling water. Leave to infuse for about 10 minutes. Strain and drink.

Heath speedwell tea is often used to relieve symptoms of colds and flu, as well as an antibacterial and anti-inflammatory aid. It may also help in treating upper respiratory tract infections.

Heath Speedwell Tincture

Ingredients:
- 200 grams of dried heath speedwell
- 1 liter of vodka or spirit

Preparation: Place the dried herb into a jar. Pour over the alcohol so that it completely covers the herb. Leave in a dark, cool place for about 2-3 weeks, stirring daily. After this time, strain the tincture and store in a dark bottle.

A heath speedwell tincture can be applied externally to the skin to reduce inflammation and accelerate wound healing. *Always use in moderation and with caution.*

Heath Speedwell Oil

Ingredients:
- 1 cup of dried heath speedwell
- 1 cup of coconut oil or olive oil

Preparation: Put the dried herb into a jar. Pour over the coconut oil or olive oil. Close the jar and place it in a warm place for about 4 weeks. Remember to shake the jar daily. After this time, strain the oil and store it in a dark bottle.

This oil is an excellent massage aid for the skin, helping to alleviate inflammation and bruises, and stimulating wound healing. It can also be used as a home remedy for dry and irritated skin..

Triterpenes: These substances are known for their anti-inflammatory and antimicrobial properties, which may help in treating skin inflammations and skin infections.

Saponins: Saponins are natural cleansers that may help clear the skin and counteract acne. They also have anti-inflammatory effects, which may help reduce redness and irritation.

Flavonoids: Flavonoids are powerful antioxidants that help protect the skin from damage caused by free radicals. They may also help promote the health and firmness of the skin.

Rosmarinic Acid: This acid is a known anti-allergic and antimicrobial agent that may aid in treating skin conditions such as eczema or psoriasis.

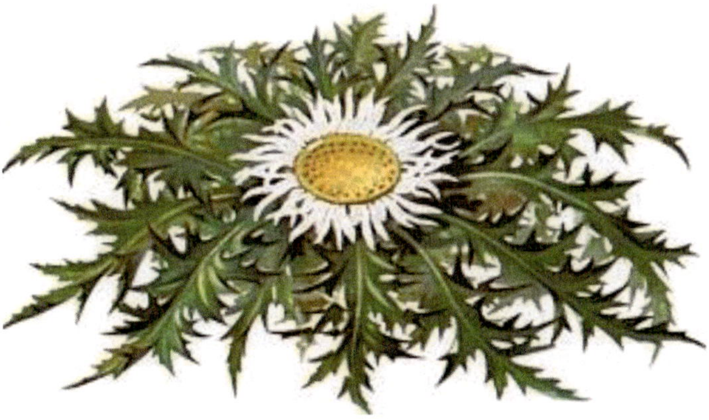

Stemless carline thistle (Carlina acaulis)

This is a plant that is traditionally used in folk medicine to alleviate digestive ailments such as indigestion and stomach pain.

Stemless Carline Thistle Infusion

Ingredients:
- 2 tablespoons of dried eyebright flowers
- 2 cups of boiling water

Preparation: Pour the boiling water into a vessel containing dried Carline thistle flowers. Leave to brew for about 10 minutes. Strain the infusion and consume 1-2 times a day.

Stemless Carline thistle infusion can be used to alleviate digestive ailments such as indigestion and stomach ache.

Stemless Carline Thistle Tincture

Ingredients:
- 100 g of dried Carline thistle flowers
- 500 ml of vodka or spirits

Preparation: Place the dried Carline thistle flowers in a glass jar. Pour in alcohol, so that it completely covers the flowers. Screw the jar and leave it in a dark place for about 2 weeks. After this time, strain the tincture and store it in a dark bottle.

Stemless Carline thistle tincture can be used to alleviate digestive ailments such as indigestion and stomach ache.

Stemless Carline Thistle Honey

Ingredients:
- 2 tablespoons of dried Carline thistle flowers
- 1 cup of honey

Preparation: In a jar, mix Carline thistle flowers with honey. Screw the jar and leave it for 2-3 weeks, stirring every day. After this time, the honey can be used by the teaspoon before meals. Stemless Carline thistle honey can be used to alleviate digestive ailments such as indigestion and stomach pain. Honey from this plant is indeed a very potent remedy, use it with moderation and sensibly.

Flavonoids: These plant compounds are known antioxidants and can help fight free radicals in the body.

Polyacetylenes: These compounds have antifungal and antibacterial effects.

Terpenoids, including karlin, karlinol, inulin: These compounds have strong anti-inflammatory and antibacterial actions.

Mineral salts: Stemless Carline thistle contains many minerals that are important for health, including potassium, calcium, magnesium, and zinc.

Organic acids: Various organic acids are present in the stemless Carline thistle, which have a beneficial impact on health, such as citric acid and malic acid.

Stemless Carline thistle, also known as the ‚flower of immortality', is a plant whose power lies in its subtle beauty and potent healing power. Its collection is a ritual that connects us with our ancestors, as well as with nature, from which we derive so much. In the flowering period, from July to September, when the sun is highest in the sky, and the plant is most saturated with life-giving ingredients, we undertake this ancient rite of gathering. This is the moment when the roots and rhizomes of the thistle are most full of their valuable active ingredients.

Selected with love and respect, the roots and rhizomes are then carefully cleaned and then dried in the shade, in a place where the breeze can gently move them, much like leaves on a tree. This process, though simple, is crucial for preserving their powerful healing properties. These dried treasures from the thistle become the basis for various preparations - from infusions, through macerates, to tinctures. These traditional preparation methods allow us to derive the full benefits of this extraordinary plant. Stemless Carline thistle is a multi-purpose plant that played a key role in the medicine of ancient peoples. It was valued for its versatile medicinal properties, especially for liver protection, supporting digestive processes, and anti-inflammatory action. It is a true gift of nature that helps us maintain balance and health in our body.

So let's immerse ourselves in this experience, exploring the mysteries of the thistle, harnessing its power and enjoying its benefits. The adventure with this plant is not only a journey to the roots of our medicine, but also the opportunity to discover new, healthier paths to live everyday life.

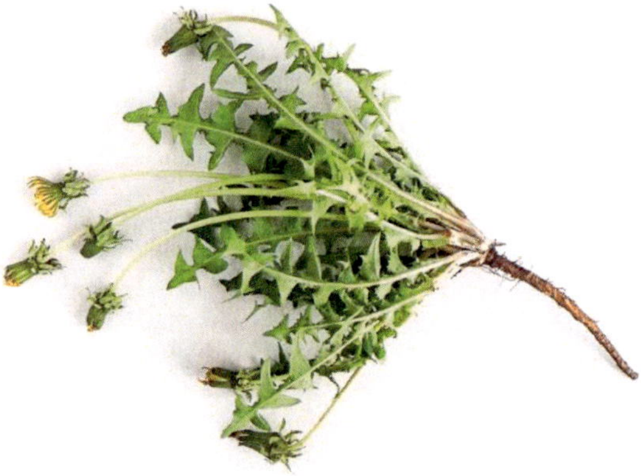

Dandelion Root (Taraxacum officinale radix)
Dandelion root is used as a cleansing and detoxifying agent, supporting the work of the liver.

Dandelion Root Infusion

Ingredients:
- 2 tablespoons of dried dandelion root
- 1 cup of water

Preparation: Put the dandelion root into a pot and pour a cup of water over it. Simmer on low heat for about 10 minutes. Remove from heat, strain, and let cool. You can drink the infusion 2-3 times a day.

A dandelion root infusion can be used as a cleansing and detoxifying agent, supporting the work of the liver.

Dandelion Root Tincture

Ingredients:

- 100 g of dried dandelion root
- 500 ml of 70% alcohol

Preparation: Place the dried dandelion root in a jar and then pour alcohol over it. Close the jar tightly and set it aside in a dark place for about 2 weeks. Shake the jar daily. After this time, strain the tincture and store in a dark bottle. Use 2-3 times a day, 20-30 drops diluted in a small amount of water.

A dandelion root tincture is used for liver problems, digestive system issues, and as a body detoxifier.

Dandelion Root Syrup

Ingredients:

- 200 g of dandelion root
- 1 l of water
- 500 g of honey

Preparation: Wash the dandelion root, cut into small pieces, and pour water over it. Simmer on low heat for about an hour. Strain, and add honey to the remaining liquid. Cook on low heat for another 30 minutes until the syrup thickens. Pour into a bottle and store in the refrigerator. Use 1-2 tablespoons a day.

Dandelion root syrup is used as a supplement to support liver function, the digestive system, and detoxify the body.

Dandelion Root Mixture

Ingredients:

- 1 tablespoon of dried dandelion root
- 1 cup of water
- 1 tablespoon of honey (optional)

Preparation: Pour a cup of hot water over the dried dandelion root and leave it to infuse for about 10-15 minutes. After this time, strain the infusion. If you wish, you can add a spoonful of honey to improve the taste. You can drink the mixture 2-3 times a day. A dandelion root mixture may help in cleansing the body and supporting liver function.

Dandelion Root Throat Rinse

Ingredients:

- 1 tablespoon of dried dandelion root
- 1 cup of water

Preparation: Pour a cup of boiling water over the dandelion root and leave it to infuse for about 15 minutes. After this time, strain the infusion. You can use the rinse to gargle 2-3 times a day.

A dandelion root rinse may provide relief for sore throats, inflammation, and infections.

Dandelion Leaf Infusion

Ingredients:

- 1 teaspoon of dried dandelion leaves
- 1 cup of boiling water

Preparation: Place the dried dandelion leaves in a cup. Pour over the boiling water and leave it to steep for about 10 minutes. Strain the infusion and it is ready to consume.

A dandelion leaf infusion may help in detoxifying the body, supporting digestion, and promoting liver and kidney function.

Vitamins: Dandelion is a good source of vitamins, including A, C, D, E, K, and B vitamins (such as B1, B2, B3, B5, B6, and B12).

Minerals It contains minerals like potassium, calcium, magnesium, iron, copper, zinc, sodium, and phosphorus.

Inulin: Dandelion root is a rich source of inulin, a type of prebiotic fiber that can support gut health.

Taraxacin: This is a bitter substance that helps stimulate appetite and improve digestion.

Dandelion also contains flavonoids, which are known antioxidants.

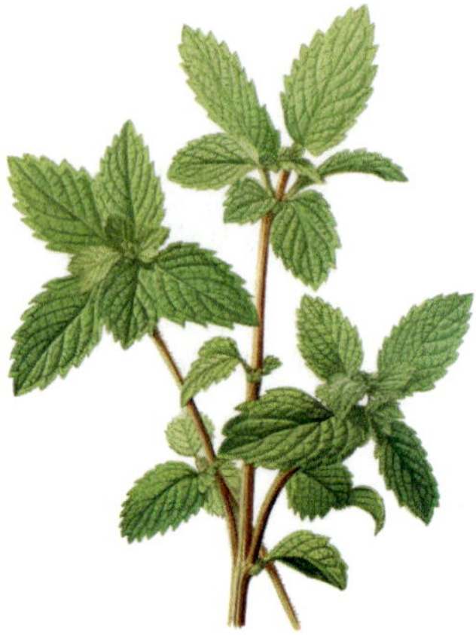

Lemon Balm (Melissa officinalis)
Lemon balm is known for its calming, antiviral, and anti-inflammatory properties.

Lemon Balm Tea

Ingredients:
- 1 łtablespoon fresh or dried lemon balm leaves
- 1 cup boiling water

Preparation: Pour the hot water over the lemon balm leaves and let it steep for 10-15 minutes. Strain and serve. The tea can be drunk 2-3 times a day. It has a calming effect, alleviates stress and tension, helps with sleep problems. It counteracts the spasms of the smooth muscles of the digestive tract, alleviates symptoms of indigestion, and promotes bile flow.

Lemon Balm Tincture

Ingredients:
- 100 g fresh lemon balm leaves
- 500 ml of spirits or vodka

Preparation: Place the lemon balm leaves in a jar, cover with spirits or vodka. Leave in a dark place for about 2 weeks, shaking the jar daily. After this time, strain the tincture and transfer it to a bottle.

Lemon balm tincture can be used externally for washing wounds, as it has antibacterial properties. Internally, it has a calming effect, reduces stress, and supports digestion.

Lemon Balm Oil

Ingredients:
- 1 cup fresh lemon balm leaves
- 1 cup of coconut oil or olive oil

Preparation: Cover the lemon balm leaves with oil in a jar. Leave in a warm, dark place for about 2 weeks, shaking the jar daily. After this time, strain the oil and store it in a dark bottle.

Lemon balm oil can be used externally on the skin. It has anti-inflammatory properties, accelerates wound healing and is helpful in treating herpes.

Lemon Balm Syrup

Ingredients:
- 2 cups fresh lemon balm leaves
- 1 cup water
- 1 cup sugar (can be replaced with honey for a healthier version).

Preparation: Place the lemon balm leaves in a pot, add water and sugar. Cook on low heat until the sugar is completely dissolved. Cook for another 10 minutes, then remove from the heat and let it cool. When the syrup has cooled, strain it and transfer it to a bottle. Store in the refrigerator.

Lemon balm syrup can be used to alleviate symptoms of cold and flu, thanks to the anti-inflammatory and antiviral properties of lemon balm. Additionally, drinking it before bedtime can help improve sleep quality.

Vitamins: Lemon balm is a good source of vitamins, such as vitamin C, which is a powerful antioxidant. It also contains several B vitamins that are essential for the proper functioning of the nervous system and metabolic processes in the body.

Minerals: Lemon balm contains minerals such as magnesium, iron, calcium, potassium, and copper.

Phenolic acids: Lemon balm contains phenolic acids, such as rosmarinic acid, which is a well-known antioxidant and antibacterial agent.

Terpeny: Lemon balm contains terpenes such as citral, citronellol, and geraniol, which give lemon balm its characteristic lemony aroma and have antiviral and anti-inflammatory effects..

Flavonoids: Flavonoids are powerful antioxidants that help protect the body against the harmful effects of free radicals.

Ursolic and oleanolic acid: These compounds have strong antiviral, antibacterial, and anti-inflammatory properties.

All these components make lemon balm widely used in natural medicine. It is primarily known for its calming properties, but it is also used to alleviate symptoms of cold and flu, improve digestion, and treat various skin problems.

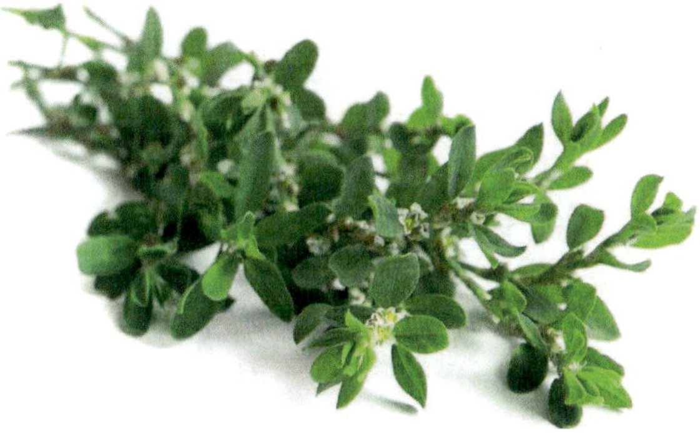

Knotweed (Polygonum aviculare)
Knotweed is used as an anti-inflammatory and antioxidant, particularly for urinary system ailments.

Knotweed infusion

Ingredients:
- 1 tablespoon of dried knotweed
- 1 cup of boiling water

Preparation: Pour the dried knotweed into a cup. Pour over with boiling water and cover. Leave to infuse for about 15 minutes. Strain.

Drinking 1-2 cups a day can help with urinary system ailments and have anti-inflammatory effects.

Urinary system issues: Due to its diuretic properties, knotweed infusion is often used to treat urinary tract infections and helps in the removal of kidney stones.

Digestive issues: Knotweed infusion can aid digestion and relieve symptoms of indigestion.

Skin problems: Thanks to its anti-inflammatory properties, knotweed infusion can be used topically to treat various skin issues, such as rashes or irritations.

Inflammation: Knotweed infusion can be taken internally to alleviate inflammation in the body, e.g. in cases of rheumatism.

Knotweed oil macerate

Ingredients:

- 1 part dried plant (in this case, dried knotweed)
- 10 part dried plant (in this case, dried knotweed)

This means that if you are using 10 grams of dried knotweed, you will need 100 ml of vegetable oil.

Preparation: Place 10 grams of dried knotweed in a jar. Add 100 ml of vegetable oil to the jar. Close the jar and mix the contents well. Place the jar in a warm, dark place for about 2-3 weeks. Shake the jar every few days to ensure that all parts of the plant are soaked in oil. After 2-3 weeks, strain the macerate through a fine sieve or cloth to remove plant residues. Pour the ready macerate into a clean, dry jar or bottle. Store in a cool, dark place.

Knotweed oil macerate can be used for moisturizing and soothing irritated skin, as well as for massage.

Flavonoids: These are powerful antioxidants that help fight against free radicals in the body. Knotweed contains many different flavonoids, including kaempferol, quercetin, and myricetin.

Phenolic acids: These are also strong antioxidants. The most important ones include chlorogenic acid, ferulic acid, and caffeic acid.

Triterpenes: These are compounds that exhibit a range of beneficial properties, including antiviral, antibacterial, and anti-inflammatory effects.
Saponins: hese are compounds that demonstrate antibacterial and antifungal actions. They may also aid in cholesterol reduction.

Vitamins and minerals: Knotweed contains a range of important vitamins and minerals, including vitamin C, calcium, magnesium, potassium, and phosphoru

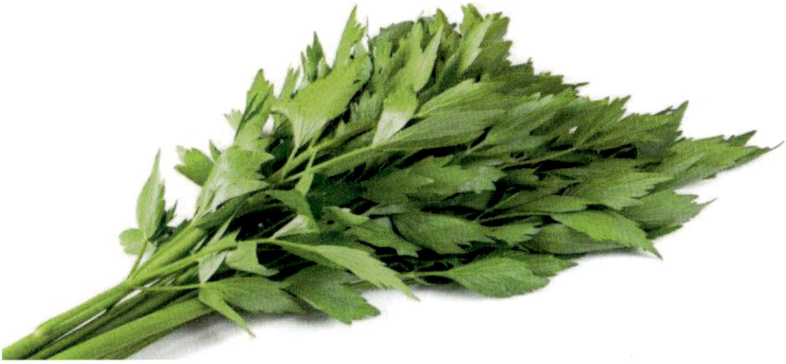

Garden Lovage (Levisticum officinale)
Lovage is used in the treatment of various ailments, such as indigestion, urinary tract infections, and also as a cough remedy.

<u>**Lovage leaf infusion**</u>

Ingredients:
- 2 teaspoons of dried lovage leaves
- 1 cup of hot water

Preparation: Pour the hot water over the dried leaves. Wait for 10 minutes and then strain. The lovage infusion is ready to consume. You can drink it 2-3 times a day, preferably after meals.

Lovage infusion can help alleviate symptoms of indigestion and urinary tract discomfort. It acts as a diuretic, which can contribute to eliminating urinary tract infections. The infusion can also soothe a cough by calming irritated respiratory passages.

Lovage Root Tincture

Ingredients:
- 100 g of lovage root
- 500 ml of spirits

Preparation: Lovage root tincture can support digestion and alleviate symptoms of indigestion. Additionally, it has a diuretic action, which can aid in treating urinary tract infections.

Lovage root tincture can support digestion and alleviate symptoms of indigestion. Additionally, it has a diuretic action, which can aid in treating urinary tract infections.

Lovage Oil

Ingredients:
- Fresh lovage leaves
- Base vegetable oil (e.g., grapeseed oil, jojoba oil)

Preparation: Pour oil over lovage leaves so that they are completely covered. Put the mixture in a jar and set aside for about 2-3 weeks in a dark place. After this time, strain the oil and store it in a dark bottle.

Lovage oil is often used in aromatherapy for its relaxing and soothing properties. It can also be used for massage, which can help alleviate muscle and joint pain. However, it's important to remember that essential oils are highly concentrated and should always be diluted before using directly on the skin

Vitamins: High content of vitamin C, which is a potent antioxidant. Lovage also contains B vitamins, including folic acid.

Minerals: High content of potassium, which is a key electrolyte responsible for regulating blood pressure. Lovage also contains magnesium, which is necessary for proper muscle and nerve function, as well as copper, iron, and calcium.

Phytonutrients: Lovage is rich in phytonutrients, such as flavonoids, which have potent antioxidant and anti-inflammatory properties.

Essential oils: Lovage contains essential oils such as eugenol, limonene, and terpenes, which have health-beneficial properties, including antibacterial, antifungal, and anti-inflammatory actions.

Quercetin Acid: This is a potent antioxidant that helps protect cells from damage. Rosmarinic Acid: It has antibacterial and anti-inflammatory actions

Remember that although lovage is a natural ingredient, it may interact with some medications and can cause allergic reactions in some individuals.

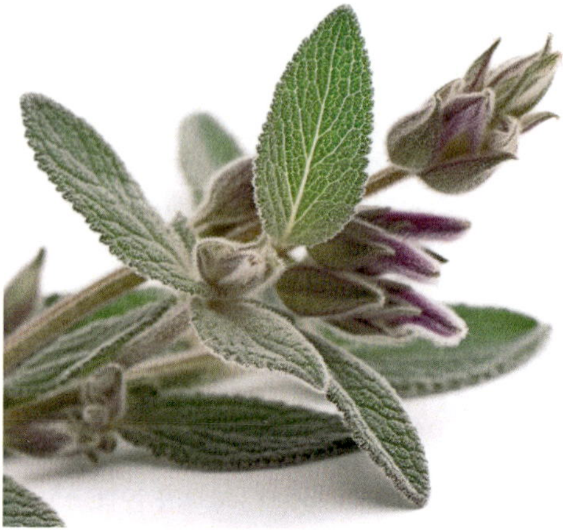

Sage (Salvia officinalis)
Sage is known for its strong antiseptic, anti-inflammatory, and antibacterial properties. Traditionally, it has been used to treat oral and throat infections

Sage Infusion

Ingredients:
- 2 teaspoons of dried sage
- 250 ml of water

Preparation: Pour hot, but not boiling, water over the dried sage and let it infuse for about 10 minutes. Strain before consumption.

A sage infusion can help alleviate throat discomfort, such as pain and inflammation. It can be consumed as a beverage, but it can also be used for gargling.

Sage Oil

Ingredients:
- 1 cup of dried sage
- 1 liter of vegetable oil (e.g., olive oil)

Preparation: Pour the dried sage with the oil into a jar. Leave for about 2-3 weeks in a dark place. After this time, strain the oil.

You can use this oil for skin massage. Sage oil is known for its anti-inflammatory and antibacterial properties.

Sage Tincture

Ingredients:
- 1 cup of dried sage
- 1 liter of alcohol

Preparation: Pour the dried sage into a jar with alcohol. Set aside for about 2-3 weeks in a dark place. After this time, strain the tincture.

Sage tincture can be used for gargling the throat and mouth in cases of infections and inflammations.

Flavonoids: This group of compounds naturally occurring in plants have strong antioxidant properties, which means they help protect our cells from harmful free radicals.

Phenolic acids: These compounds also have strong antioxidant properties. They are also anti-inflammatory and can aid in protecting the cardiovascular system.

Thujones: These are compounds naturally occurring in sage that have strong antiseptic properties. This is one of the reasons why sage is so frequently used in the treatment of oral infections.

Camphor and cineole: These are compounds that exhibit antibacterial and antifungal actions.

Vitamins and minerals: Sage is a good source of vitamins such as vitamin C, thiamine (B1), riboflavin (B2), niacin (B3), pyridoxine (B6), folate (B9), and vitamin E.

Minerals: In sage, we can find magnesium, zinc, calcium, iron, copper, and manganese.

Rosmarinic acid: This compound belongs to the group of polyphenols, which is a strong antioxidant and has antiviral activity.

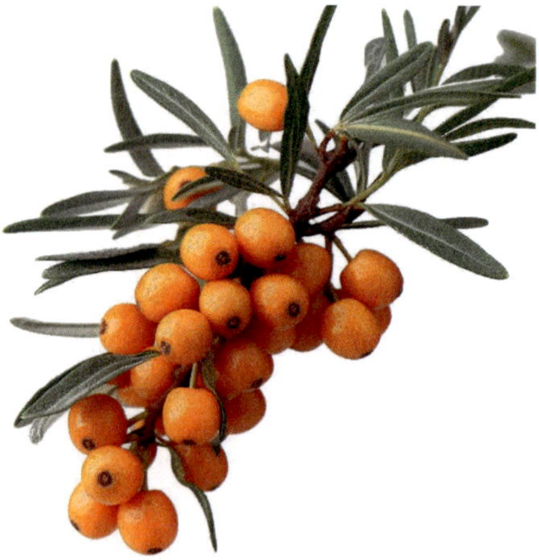

Sea Buckthorn (Hippophae rhamnoides)
Sea buckthorn is exceptionally rich in vitamins, and its fruits are used to boost immunity, regenerate skin, and protect against free radicals.

Sea Buckthorn Seed Oil

Ingredients:
- Sea buckthorn seeds
- Vegetable oil (e.g., sunflower oil, grapeseed oil) of desired concentration

A ratio of about 1:1 is recommended.
That is, if you're using 1 cup of sea buckthorn seeds, you should use about 1 cup of vegetable oil. Nevertheless, it's important that the seeds are completely covered with oil during maceration. If the seeds are not fully submerged, add more oil. After maceration and straining, the seeds can be squeezed to extract as much oil as possible.

Preparation: Grind the sea buckthorn seeds in a coffee grinder or a similar machine. Transfer them to a jar and cover with oil. Close the jar and leave it in a dark place for 2-3 weeks. After this time, strain the oil through a fine sieve or cheesecloth.

Sea buckthorn seed oil can be applied externally to the skin for regeneration and moisturization. It can also be used as an addition to salads and other dishes.

Sea Buckthorn Fruit Syrup

Ingredients:
- 1 kg of ripe sea buckthorn fruits
- 1 kg of sugar
- 1 liter of water

Preparation: Wash, dry, and transfer the sea buckthorn fruits to a pot. Add sugar and water, cook on low heat for about 1 hour. Strain through a sieve, pour into clean bottles. Store in a cool place.

Sea buckthorn fruit syrup can be added to tea, yogurts, or desserts. It is rich in vitamin C and boosts the immune system.

Sea Buckthorn Honey

Ingredients:
- 1 kg of ripe sea buckthorn fruits
- 1 kg of honey

Preparation: Wash, dry, and transfer the sea buckthorn fruits to a jar. Pour honey over them and mix well. Store in a dark place for about 2 weeks.

Sea buckthorn honey has antioxidant, strengthening, and regenerative properties. It can be used as an addition to tea or desserts.

Sea Buckthorn Leaf Tea

Ingredients:
- Fresh or dried sea buckthorn leavese rokitnika
- Hot water

Preparation: Pour hot, but not boiling, water (about 80 degrees Celsius) over the leaves. Let it steep for about 5-10 minutes. Strain and serve.

Sea buckthorn leaf tea has anti-inflammatory properties and may help strengthen the immune system.

Sea Buckthorn Fruit Juice

Ingredients:
- 1 kg of ripe sea buckthorn fruits
- 1-2 cups of water
- Sugar or honey to taste (optional)

Preparation: Wash, dry, and transfer the fruits to a juicer. Add water and extract the juice. If you wish, you can add sugar or honey to taste.

Sea buckthorn juice is rich in vitamins and antioxidants, which can help strengthen the immune system and improve overall health.

Sea Buckthorn Jam

Ingredients:
- 1 kg of ripe sea buckthorn fr
- 1 kg of sugar
- Juice of one lemon

Preparation: Wash, dry and transfer the fruits to a pot. Add sugar and lemon juice, cook on low heat for about 1 hour, until the fruits break down and a thick mass is formed. Transfer the hot jam to clean jars.

Sea buckthorn jam can be used as a spread for sandwiches, cakes, and other desserts.

Sea Buckthorn Fruit Preserve

Ingredients:
- 1 kg of fresh sea buckthorn fruits
- 1 kg of sugar
- 1 cup of water

Preparatione: Place the sea buckthorn fruits, sugar, and water in a large pot. Cook over medium heat, stirring occasionally, until the sugar dissolves. Reduce heat to medium-low and cook until the mixture thickens to a preserve consistency. This can take from 30 minutes to 1 hour. Transfer the hot preserve into sterilized jars, leaving about 1 cm of space at the top. Seal the jars and leave them to cool.

Sea buckthorn fruit preserve is an excellent addition to toasts, yogurts, or cakes. Thanks to its high vitamin content, it's a healthy alternative to traditional jams. *Remember that sea buckthorn has a strong, specific taste that might not be to everyone' s liking.*

It strengthens the immune system: Sea buckthorn is very rich in vitamin C, it contains much more of it than lemons or kiwi. Vitamin C is essential for the proper functioning of the immune system, and its regular intake can help prevent many diseases.

Improves skin condition: Sea buckthorn seed oil is rich in Omega-7 fatty acids, which are extremely important for skin health. Regular use can improve skin hydration, accelerate wound healing, and help in the treatment of skin conditions suc

Support for the circulatory system: Sea buckthorn also contains large amounts of flavonoids, which are powerful antioxidants. Research has shown that they can help protect against heart disease, by preventing damage caused by free radicals and reducing inflammation.

Support for the digestive system: Sea buckthorn fruits can help in the treatment of various digestive ailments, such as constipation or stomach ulcers. They are a rich source of fiber, which is essential for the health of the digestive system.

Vision protection: Sea buckthorn contains a large amount of carotenoids, which are important for eye health. They can help prevent some forms of age-related vision loss, such as cataracts or macular degeneration.

Vitamins: Sea buckthorn is exceptionally rich in vitamin C - its fruits contain much more of it than lemons. It also contains B group vitamins (B1, B2, B6, B9), vitamin E, which is a strong antioxidant, as well as vitamins A and K.

Minerals: Sea buckthorn contains many minerals, including potassium, calcium, magnesium, iron, copper, manganese, selenium, and zinc.

Fatty acids: Sea buckthorn is one of the few plant sources of omega-7 acid, which is extremely beneficial for skin health. It also contains omega-3 and omega-6 acids, which are important for heart health.

Flavonoids: Sea buckthorn fruits are rich in flavonoids, which are powerful antioxidants and can help protect against heart disease and certain types of cancer.

Carotenoids: Sea buckthorn contains a large amount of carotenoids, which are important for eye and skin health.

Protein: Sea buckthorn fruits also contain protein, which is quite rare among fruits.

Fiber: Sea buckthorn is a source of fiber, which helps regulate the digestive system. Phenolic compounds: Sea buckthorn contains numerous phenolic compounds, which demonstrate strong antioxidant activity.

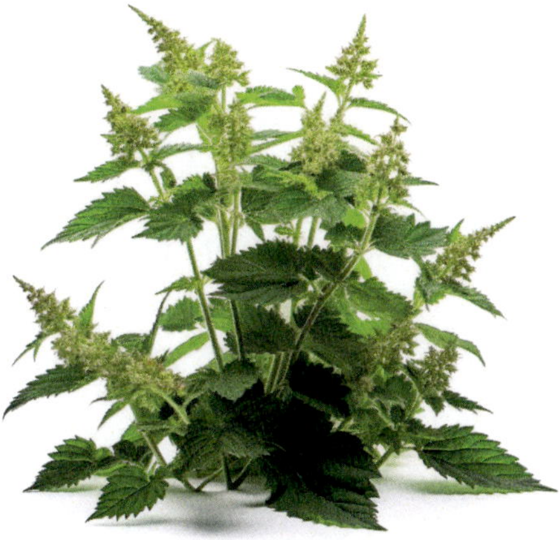

Stinging Nettle (Urtica urens)
Nettle is a potent detoxifying agent, it aids in the treatment of urinary tract infections and improves the overall condition of the body.

Nettle infusion

Ingredients:
- 1 tablespoon dried nettle leaves
- 1 cup of hot water

Preparation: Pour hot water over the dried nettle leaves. Cover and leave to infuse for about 10 minutes. Strain and serve warm.

Nettle infusion is recommended for body detoxification and support of the urinary system.

Nettle Juice

Ingredients:
- A handful of fresh nettle leaves
- 1 cup of water

Preparation: Wash the nettle leaves, then throw them into a blender. Add water and blend until smooth. Strain through a fine sieve or cheesecloth to remove leaf residues.

Nettle juice is a real health booster. It can be drunk on an empty stomach to improve digestion and detoxify the body.

Nettle Oil Macerate

Ingredients:
- Fresh nettle leaves
- Vegetable oil (e.g. grape seed oil)

Preparation: Wash and dry the nettle leaves, then throw them into a jar. Pour oil over the leaves so that they are completely covered. Close the jar tightly and leave it in a dark, cool place for about 6 weeks. After this time, strain the oil and store it in a dark place.

Nettle oil macerate is excellent for skin care, especially for problems such as acne, psoriasis, or eczema. Apply it topically to problematic skin areas.

Vitamins: Nettle contains large amounts of vitamin C, which has strong antioxidant properties, as well as B vitamins, which are essential for the proper functioning of the nervous system. It also contains vitamin K, which is necessary for proper blood clotting and bone health, as well as beta-carotene, which is a precursor of vitamin A.

Minerals: Nettle is rich in minerals such as iron, which is necessary for the production of red blood cells, magnesium, which helps in muscle function, and calcium, which is necessary for the health of bones and teeth. It also contains potassium, copper, zinc, and selenium.

Other substances: Nettle also contains many other biologically active substances, such as polyphenols (including flavonoids), which have strong antioxidant and anti-inflammatory properties. It also contains sterols, lectins, and chlorophyll.

Protein: Nettle is also a good source of protein, which is extremely rare for green plants.

Fiber: Nettle is also rich in fiber, which is necessary for the proper functioning of the digestive system.

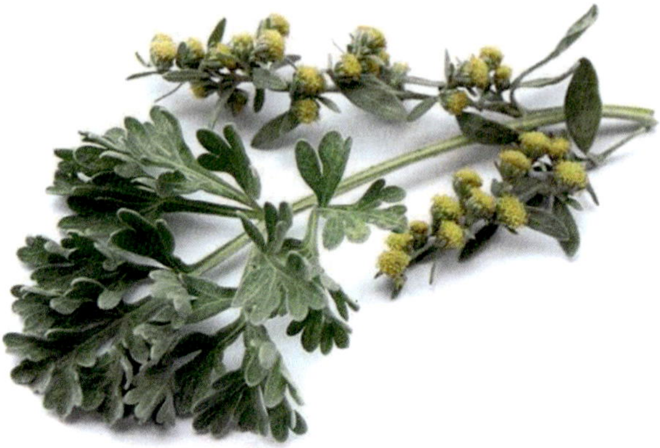

Wormwood (Artemisia absinthium)
Wormwood was traditionally used as an antiparasitic agent, as well as to aid digestion and alleviate pain.

<u>Wormwood Infusion</u>

Ingredients
- 1 teaspoon dried wormwood
- 1 cup boiling water

Preparation: Pour boiling water over the dried wormwood leaves and let it steep for about 10-15 minutes. Strain the infusion and consume in small sips. Do not exceed a dose of 2-3 cups per day.

A wormwood infusion is used to improve digestion and alleviate stomach pains. Its antiparasitic properties can also be used to combat some types of parasites.

Tincture of Wormwood

Ingredients
- 100 g dried wormwood
- 500 ml alcohol (e.g., spirit)

Preparation: Put wormwood in a glass jar, then pour alcohol over it. Leave it in a dark place for about 2 weeks, stirring daily. After this time, strain the liquid and store it in a dark bottle.

Wormwood tincture is used as an antiparasitic and antiviral agent. It can also be used to improve digestion and alleviate stomach pains. The tincture is taken orally, diluting a few drops in a glass of water.

Wormwood Ointment

Ingredients
- 2 tablespoons dried wormwood leaves
- 1/2 cup coconut oil
- 1/4 scup beeswax

Preparation: Boil the coconut oil in a saucepan, then add the dried wormwood leaves. Reduce the heat to low and heat for about 2 hours, stirring occasionally. Then add the beeswax to this and heat until it melts. After this time, strain the mixture through a tightly woven cloth or gauze into a clean jar. Leave the ointment to cool and harden.

Wormwood ointment can be applied topically to the skin to alleviate inflammation and muscle pains.

It also has antiparasitic effects. *Wormwood is a powerful plant and should be used with caution. It is not recommended for pregnant and breastfeeding women, people with liver and kidney diseases, and children.*

Bitter compounds: These compounds, called absinthin, are responsible for the characteristic bitter taste of wormwood. They stimulate the production of bile and digestive enzymes, which accelerates digestion and aids in the treatment of indigestion.

Flavonoids: These powerful antioxidants help protect the body from the harmful effects of free radicals.

Thujones: Thujones have strong antiparasitic, antibacterial, and antifungal actions.

Phenols: They have antibacterial, anti-inflammatory, and antiviral properties.

Vitamins and minerals: Wormwood contains small amounts of vitamins, such as vitamin C and some B vitamins, as well as minerals such as magnesium, zinc, and potassium.

Wormwood, a valuable ingredient in ancient and contemporary herbal medicine, is known for its strong antiparasitic and digestive actions. Its intense, bitter taste has for centuries served as a stimulant for the digestive system, aiding in alleviating many ailments such as indigestion, bloating, or lack of appetite.

However, its use extends far beyond the digestive system - wormwood is also used in the treatment of gynecological ailments and as an aid in alleviating symptoms of depression.
This universal, but often underrated ingredient of the herbal medicine cabinet, is a great example of how the past, present, and future of medicine can meet in one, unassuming plant.

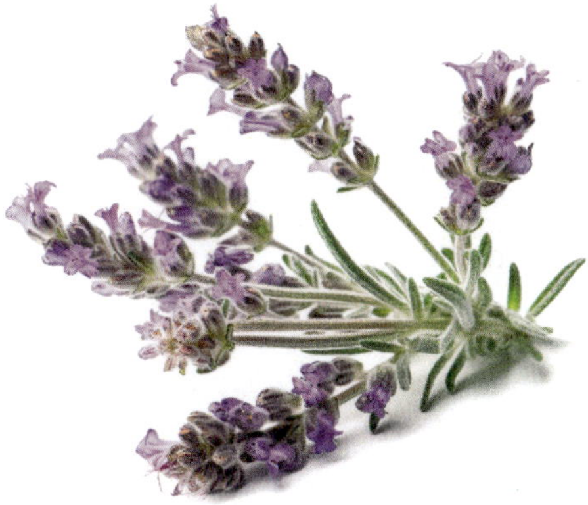

Lavender (Lavandula officinalis)
Lavender is widely known for its relaxing and calming properties. It is often used in the treatment of insomnia, anxiety disorders, and muscle tension.

Lavender Essential Oil

Ingredients:
- Lavender (fresh flowers)
- Coconut or Grape Seed Oil

Preparation: Place fresh lavender flowers in a jar. Cover the flowers with any oil (e.g. grape seed oil, coconut oil). Close the jar and leave it in a warm place for about 3-6 weeks.
After this time, strain the oil through a fine sieve or cheesecloth.

Lavender essential oil is very versatile. It can be used for massages, for baths, as an addition to creams and ointments, as well as in aromatherapy.

Lavender Tea

Ingredients:

- 1-2 teaspoons of dried lavende
- 1 scup of boiling water

Preparation: Pour boiling water over dried lavender flowers. Allow to brew for about 10 minutes, then strain.

Lavender tea is known for its relaxing and calming properties. It helps with sleep problems and alleviates stress.

Lavender Honey

Ingredients:

- Dried lavender flowers
- Natural honey

Preparation: Add dried lavender flowers to a jar. Pour honey over and mix well. Leave for 2 weeks, stirring every few days.
After this time, you can strain the honey through a fine sieve, if you prefer, but it is not necessary.

Lavender honey is an excellent addition to tea or desserts.
Lavender gives it a unique, aromatic flavor.

Lavender Ointment

Ingredients:

- 1/2 cup of coconut oil
- 2 tablespoons of dried lavender flowers
- 1/4 cup of beeswax
- 5-10 drops of lavender essential oil (optional, for a stronger aroma)

Preparation: In a saucepan, heat the coconut oil and lavender flowers over medium heat, stirring every few minutes. Do not allow it to boil - heat for about 30 minutes to allow the flowers to release their oils into the coconut oil. After heating, strain the oil through a fine sieve or cheesecloth to remove the flowers.

To the strained oil, add beeswax. Heat on low, stirring until the wax completely melts. If using, add drops of lavender essential oil and mix. Pour the mixture into small jars or ointment tins. Allow it to cool and solidify.

Lavender ointment soothes the skin, helps with burns, insect bites, dry skin, or minor wounds. It's also a great, natural lip balm.

Terpenes: Lavender contains plant terpenes such as linalool and linalyl acetate, which have anti-inflammatory, antibacterial, and antiviral effects.

Flavonoids: These compounds have strong antioxidant activity, which helps protect the body's cells from harmful free radical damage.

Coumarins: These substances have anti-inflammatory and antibacterial effects.

Minerals: Lavender contains various minerals such as calcium, iron, copper, and manganese.

Vitamins: It also contains vitamins, including vitamin A (supports skin and eye health) and some from the B vitamin group, which are essential for the proper functioning of the nervous system.

Fatty Acids: Lavender contains small amounts of fatty acids, which are beneficial for skin health and the circulatory system.

Polyphenols: These plant compounds have strong antioxidant properties and may help protect the body against various diseases.

As befits a herbalist, I would like to draw attention to the specific properties of lavender. Lavender, the lady of the herb garden, most often reveals her medicinal attributes through intensely fragrant essential oil. However, it is highly concentrated, which carries the need to use it with respect and caution.

Absolutely, lavender, although wonderful, is not for everyone - some people may experience an allergic reaction. Therefore, I always recommend testing the reaction on a small area of skin before full application of this aromatic gift of nature. Safety and well-being are key, even in the herbal world.

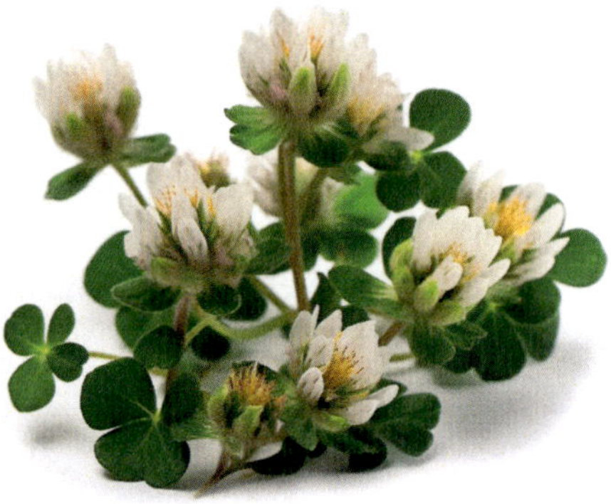

White Clover (Trifolium repens)

White clover has anti-inflammatory and soothing properties, often used to treat skin ailments, and high phytohormone content.

<u>White Clover Infusion</u>

Ingredients:

- 2 tablespoons dried white clover flowers
- 2 cups of water

Preparation: Pour boiling water over the clover flowers and leave to infuse for about 15 minutes. Strain. You can drink 2-3 times a day.

This infusion can help alleviate menopause symptoms and support skin health.

White Clover Ointment

Ingredients:
- 1 cup dried white clover flowers
- 1 cup coconut oil
- 1/4 cup beeswax

Preparation: In a pot over low heat, melt coconut oil and beeswax. When the ingredients are combined, add clover flowers and simmer on low for about 1 hour, stirring frequently. Then strain the mixture through a cheesecloth into a clean jar, let it cool down.

This ointment can be applied to the skin to soothe inflammation.

White Clover Tincture

Ingredients:
- 1 cup fresh white clover flowers
- 2 cups high-quality vodka (or another neutral spirit)

Preparation: Place the flowers in a jar and cover with alcohol, making sure all the flowers are completely covered. Close the jar and store it in a dark, cool place for about 4-6 weeks, shaking the jar daily. After this time, strain the tincture through cheesecloth and store in a dark bottle.

White clover tincture can be used to alleviate menopause and PMS symptoms.

Typically, 2-3 ml of tincture is used 2-3 times a day, but this dosage may vary depending on individual needs and body reactions.

White Clover Flower Tea

Ingredients:
- 2 tablespoons fresh white clover flowers (or 1 tablespoon dried)
- 1 cup boiling water

Preparation: Put the clover flowers in a teapot or cup. Pour boiling water and let it steep under a lid for about 10-15 minutes to ensure a good infusion. After this time, strain the infusion and if necessary, add honey to taste.

White clover flower tea is known for its soothing and anti-inflammatory properties, as well as supporting properties during menopause. It can be consumed 2-3 times a day.

Vitamins: Vitamin C: An antioxidant supporting immunity and skin health. B Vitamins: Support the functioning of the nervous system and metabolism.

Minerals: Calcium: Important for the health of bones and teeth. Magnesium: Helps in the functioning of muscles and the nervous system.

Iron: Essential for the production of red blood cells. Isoflavones: Plant phytohormones with estrogen-like activity, which can have an impact on hormonal regulation.

Kaempferol is also present in many clover species. This is a type of flavonoid with potential anti-inflammatory and antioxidant properties.

White clover, this recognizable plant with white, spherical inflorescences, is not only a charming landscape element but also a treasury of health benefits. In antiquity, both among the Vikings and other European peoples, it was respected for its medicinal powers. The Vikings, who knew the application of this plant by heart, used it to treat many ailments. They were the first to discover that the root of this plant is a powerful component that allows for blood purification, energy boost, and combating respiratory ailments.

However, it was not just the root that had its magical properties. The leaves of clover, rich in phytoestrogens, were valued as a means of regulating hormonal balance, especially among women. The Holy Grail of natural treatment, as white clover was called, is not just ancient beliefs. Modern scientific research confirms its powerful anti-inflammatory, antioxidant, and detoxifying action. These remarkable properties of white clover deserve attention so that we can benefit from its blessings, while respecting it as an essential part of our ecosystem.

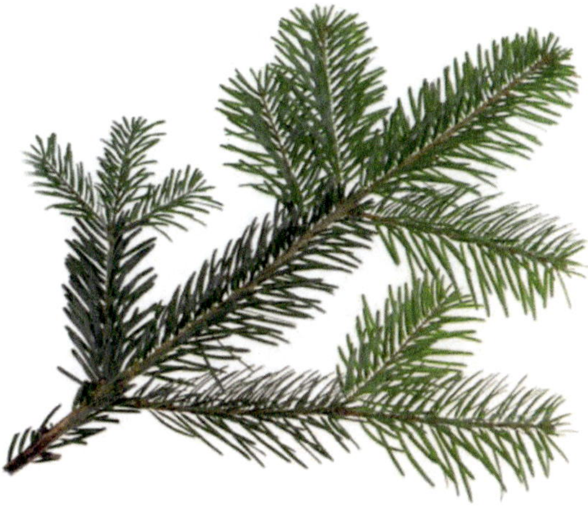

European Silver Fir (Abies albaa)
Silver fir needles are a source of essential oil with strong antiseptic properties. They are used in the treatment of respiratory tract infections.

<u>**Silver Fir Needle Tea**</u>

Ingredients:
- 1 handful of fresh silver fir needles
- 1 liter of water

Preparation: Wash the fir needles and gently crush them. Pour water into a pot and bring it to a boil. Add fir needles to the boiling water and simmer on low heat for about 10 minutes. Strain the infusion and consume it hot. You can add honey to taste.

The tea primarily acts on the respiratory system - it soothes cough, aids in mucus secretion, and alleviates symptoms of asthma. It also contains antioxidants, which help fight free radicals in the body, counteracting aging processes.

Silver Fir Needle Syrup

Ingredients:

- 5-7 handfuls of fresh silver fir needles
- 1 liter of watery
- 500 g of sugar

Preparation: Wash the fir needles and gently crush them. Pour water into a pot and bring it to a boil. Add fir needles to the boiling water and simmer on low heat for about 10 minutes. Add sugar and simmer on low heat, stirring, until the sugar dissolves and the syrup begins to thicken. Strain the syrup and pour it into sterilized bottles. Store in a cool, dark place.

The syrup has similar benefits for the respiratory system as the tea but is more concentrated and sweeter. It can be especially useful for people with sore throats or coughs. Additionally, thanks to the sugar content, it provides extra energy.

Vitamins: Fir needles are particularly rich in vitamin C, which is a strong antioxidant, and also contain vitamin A, which is beneficial for eye and skin health.

Minerals: Fir needles also contain various minerals, such as potassium, calcium, and magnesium, which are necessary for bone health and the nervous system.

Phenolic Compounds: These compounds have strong antioxidant properties and may help protect the body from the harmful effects of free radicals.

Terpeny: These compounds have strong antioxidant properties and can help protect the body from the harmful effects of free radicals.

Flavonoids: These are plant compounds with powerful antioxidant properties that can help protect against heart disease and some types of cancer.

Although often overlooked, fir needles hide health secrets that have been appreciated for centuries by the peoples inhabiting the forests of Europe. They, known for their unique, forest aroma, were used as raw materials for making nutritious infusions and oils that protected health and strengthened vitality. For the ancient Vikings and other Scandinavian tribes, fir needles were a symbol of longevity and courage. They believed that their power penetrated into the infusion, giving it strength for body and spirit.

In folk medicine, fir needles were used to treat various ailments, from coughs and colds, to respiratory problems and rheumatism. Today, this knowledge is revived thanks to scientific research confirming these ancient beliefs. Essential oils contained in fir needles, such as limonene, bornyl acetate, and pinene, show strong antibacterial, anti-inflammatory, and antifungal activity. Therefore, fir needles can be a valuable support in fighting various infections and alleviating pain symptoms.

So I invite you on a journey to the heart of the forest, to the world of fir, where at every step you can discover its power and benefits. This experience will help us understand how valuable these green needles, which we can encounter on our way, are and how much they can bring to our health. After all, they are the treasure of our natural medicine, waiting to be discovered.

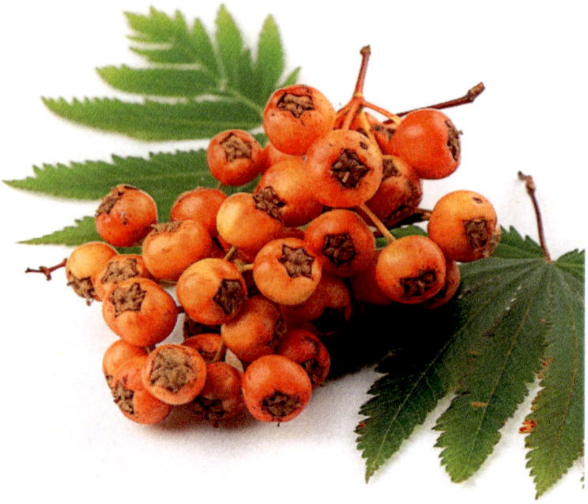

Rowan (Sorbus aucuparia)
Rowan fruits are rich in vitamin C and have anti-inflammatory properties. They are used in the treatment of upper respiratory tract infections.

Recipe for Rowan Jam

Ingredients:
- 1 kg of ripe rowan fruitsy
- 1 kg of sugar
- Juice of 1 lemon

Preparation: Wash the rowan thoroughly, then drain and remove all stalks. Transfer the fruits to a pot, add sugar and lemon juice. Cook over medium heat until the fruits soften and the sugar completely dissolves. Transfer the hot jam to sterile jars, close tightly, and turn upside down to cool.

Rowan jam is rich in vitamin C and can be used as a home remedy to boost immunity, especially during the autumn-winter period.

Rowan Liqueur Recipe

Ingredients:
- 1 kg of ripe rowan fruits
- 1 liter of vodka
- 500 g of sugar

Preparation: Wash the rowan, drain and remove the stalks. Transfer the fruits to a large jar, add sugar and vodka. Close the jar tightly and set aside in a dark, cool place for 2-3 months. Shake the liqueur gently every few days. After this time, strain the liqueur through a closely woven cloth and transfer to bottles.

Rowan liqueur is valued for its health properties, especially during the cold season. It has anti-inflammatory and immune-boosting effects. It can be used as a home remedy for colds and flu.

Infusion of Rowan Fruits

Ingredients:
- 2 tablespoons of ripe rowan fruits
- 1 cup of boiling water

Preparation: Pour boiling water over the ripe rowan fruits and leave to infuse for about 10 minutes. Strain the infusion and drink 2-3 times a day.

Rowan Fruit Syrup

Ingredients:
- 1 kg of rowan fruits
- 1 kg of sugar
- 1 liter of water

Preparation: Rinse the rowan fruits, dry them and put them in a large pot. Add sugar and water, then cook over medium heat for about 1 hour. When the syrup starts to thicken, remove it from the heat and strain it through a sieve or dense gauze. Pour the ready syrup into sterilized bottles and close.

The syrup is an excellent addition to tea, especially during the cold and flu season.

Rowan Leaf Infusion

Ingredients:
- A handful of dried rowan leaves
- 1 cup of boiling water

Preparation: Pour boiling water over dried rowan leaves and brew for about 10 minutes. After this time, strain the infusion. Rowan leaf infusion is traditionally used to soothe sore throats and aid in the treatment of upper respiratory tract infections.

Remember to wash rowanberries thoroughly before eating them and it's best to cook them a bit as they may contain small amounts of toxins, which are removed in the cooking process.

Vitamins: Rowan is particularly rich in vitamin C, which is a strong antioxidant, strengthens the immune system, and helps fight infections. It also contains B vitamins, which are necessary for the proper functioning of the nervous system and for metabolism.

Minerals: Rowan fruits contain various minerals such as potassium, calcium, magnesium, iron, and zinc. These minerals are important for bone health, proper muscle function, and overall health and good physical condition of the body.

Flavonoids and phenols: Rowan is rich in bioactive compounds such as flavonoids and phenols, which are strong antioxidants and can help protect against various diseases, including heart disease and some types of cancer.

Fiber: Rowan fruits are also a source of fiber, which helps regulate the digestive system and may contribute to maintaining a healthy body weight.

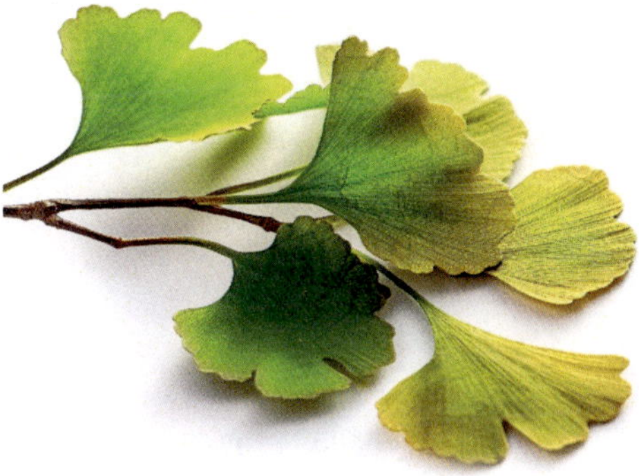

Ginkgo biloba (Ginkgo biloba)
It is a unique plant species that has survived on Earth unchanged since prehistoric times. Commonly known as the „maidenhair tree", this extraordinary plant is a symbol of endurance and longevity.

Its valuable leaves, which turn golden in the autumn, are prized for their potent medicinal properties.

They are used worldwide in natural medicine to improve memory and concentration. The main active compounds found in Ginkgo biloba leaves are flavonoids and terpenoids, known for their strong antioxidant action.

Tea made from Ginkgo biloba leaves

Ingredients:
- 1-2 teaspoons of dried Ginkgo biloba leaves
- 1 cup of hot water

Preparation: Pour hot water over the dried leaves and brew for about 10 minutes. After this time, strain and allow the tea to cool down. You can drink it 1-2 times a day.

Ginkgo biloba tea is used to improve memory and concentration, it may also support blood circulation.

Ginkgo Biloba Tincture

Ingredients:
- 1 cup of dried Ginkgo biloba leaves
- 1 liter of spirits

Preparation: Place the Ginkgo biloba leaves in a large jar, then pour over the spirits. Leave the jar in a dark, cool place for about 4 weeks. After this time, strain the tincture and store in dark bottles.

The Ginkgo biloba tincture can be used internally to improve memory and concentration, as well as to support blood circulation. The recommended dose is 1-2 teaspoons per day.

Ginkgo Biloba Oil

Ingredients:
- 1 cup of dried Ginkgo biloba leaves
- 2 cups of vegetable oil (for example coconut oil or olive oil)

Preparation: Place the Ginkgo biloba leaves in a large jar, then pour over the vegetable oil. Close the jar and leave it for about 4 weeks in a dark, cool place, shaking it daily. After this time, strain the oil and store in a dark bottle.

Ginkgo biloba oil can be applied externally to the skin, for example for massages. It has properties that improve blood circulation, which can help alleviate symptoms such as cold hands and feet. It can also support skin health by improving blood circulation in the epidermis.

Ginkgo Biloba Cream

Ingredients:

- 1/2 cup of dried Ginkgo biloba leaves
- 1 cup of vegetable oil (e.g., coconut oil, jojoba oil)
- 1/4 cup of beeswax

Preparation: Grind the dried Ginkgo biloba leaves in a coffee grinder or blender. Transfer the ground leaves to a jar and pour over the vegetable oil. Close the jar and leave it in a dark place for 2-3 weeks, shaking it daily. After this time, strain the oil through a dense sieve or cheesecloth. Melt the beeswax in a water bath. Add the strained Ginkgo biloba oil to the melted beeswax, stirring to achieve a uniform consistency. Pour the cream into clean cosmetic containers and leave to cool.

Ginkgo biloba cream can be applied to the skin to improve blood circulation and oxygenate the skin. It may help to alleviate symptoms such as tired legs, swollen legs, and also to improve the appearance of the skin.

Flavonoids: This is a group of potent antioxidants that can help protect the body's cells from damage caused by free radicals.

Terpenes (terpene lactones): Two types are present in Ginkgo biloba: ginkgolides and bilobalides. Both have strong anti-inflammatory and neuroprotective properties.

Glycolic acid: Although it can cause allergic reactions in some people, glycolic acid has potent anti-inflammatory and antioxidant properties.

Minerals and vitamins: Although Ginkgo biloba is not particularly known for its high content of vitamins and minerals, it contains a certain amount of magnesium, calcium, potassium, and phosphorus.

Ginkgo leaves help to improve blood circulation, especially in the blood vessels of the brain, which directly affects cognitive abilities. For this reason, Ginkgo biloba is often used in the treatment and prevention of various memory-related conditions, such as dementia and Alzheimer's disease.

In addition, Ginkgo biloba is also used to treat problems associated with insufficient blood circulation in the legs, a condition known as peripheral artery disease.

It is also used to treat conditions such as dizziness, ringing in the ears, vision disorders, and other problems associated with damage to blood vessels and nerves.

Even though Ginkgo biloba is natural, it's always important to approach it with caution.

Some individuals may experience side effects, such as headaches, gastrointestinal disturbances, or allergic reactions.

It's always necessary to consult a doctor before starting any supplementation, especially if you are taking any prescription medications.

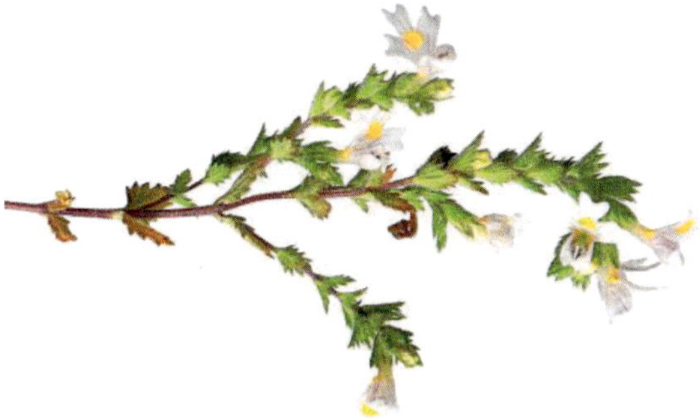

Eyebright (Euphrasia rostkoviana)
Eyebright is often used in the treatment of eye ailments, such as conjunctivitis or eye fatigue.

Eyebright Infusion

Ingredients:
- 1 teaspoon of dried eyebright
- 1 cup of boiling water

Preparation: Pour boiling water over the dried herbs and leave it covered for about 10-15 minutes. Then strain the infusion.

Use it to wash your eyes 2-3 times a day in case of eye irritation or conjunctivitis.

Eyebright Compresses

Ingredients:
- A handful of dried eyebright flowers
- 1 cup of boiling water

Preparation: Pour boiling water over the dried eyebright flowers and leave it to infuse for about 15 minutes. Then strain and cool to room temperature.

Soak a clean cotton pad in the infusion and apply to your eyes. Leave the compress on for about 10 minutes. Apply 1-2 times a day.

Tired Eyes: Regular use of compresses can help reduce feelings of fatigue and tiredness in the eyes.

Conjunctivitis: Due to its anti-inflammatory action, eyebright can help alleviate the symptoms of conjunctivitis.

Eye Infections: Eyebright has antibacterial properties, making it effective in treating eye infections.

Allergies: Compresses from this plant may provide relief from eye allergy symptoms, such as itching, burning, and redness.

Flavonoids: These are powerful antioxidants that can help protect the eyes from oxidative damage.

Iridoids: These are compounds that exhibit strong anti-inflammatory and antibacterial actions, which can be especially beneficial in treating eye infections.

Triterpenes: These are compounds that show antiviral and antiparasitic actions.

Vitamins and Minerals: Eyebright contains various vitamins, including vitamins A, C, D, and E, as well as various minerals, including potassium, magnesium, and calcium.

Eyebright (Euphrasia rostkoviana) is one of the most important herbs in traditional natural medicine, which for centuries has been a key ingredient in the treatment of eye ailments. It is valued for its unique properties, especially in the context of treating conjunctivitis, eye fatigue or even glaucoma.

The Latin name of eyebright, „Euphrasia", comes from the Greek word „euphrosyne", which means joy or gratitude. This is a direct reflection of the relief effect that this small but powerful plant provides. Eyebright contains various compounds, such as flavonoids, tannins, and iridoids, which exhibit strong anti-inflammatory and antibacterial properties.

Thanks to them, eyebright is capable of effectively alleviating irritations, redness, and swelling of the eyes. Despite advances in medicine and technology, eyebright remains a valuable ingredient in phytotherapy.

Extracts from this plant often find use in various types of eye preparations, such as drops or ointments. When our eyes are daily exposed to constant strain, such as working on a computer, eyebright is an important tool that can help maintain the health of our eyes.

Eyebright is an example of how ancient knowledge and natural treatment methods can still play a key role in maintaining our health and well-being in today's times.

Drawing on this wisdom, this humble plant, full of power, is still used by contemporary herbalists, showing that true healing can come straight from the heart of nature.

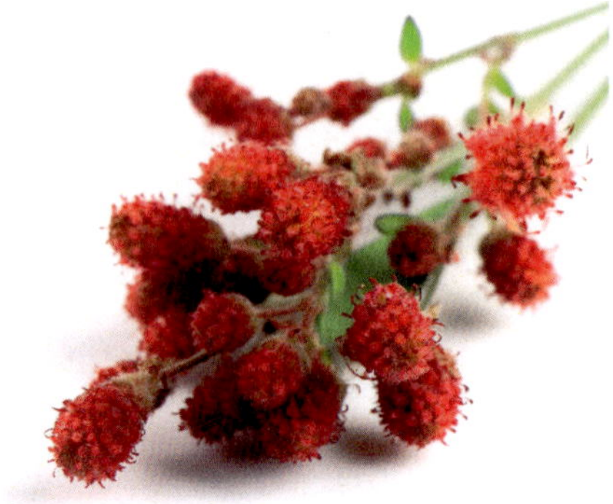

Great Burnet (Sanguisorba officinalis)
Great Burnet has hemostatic and anti-inflammatory properties, and is often used to treat wounds and inflammatory skin conditions.

<u>Great Burnet Infusion</u>

Ingredients:
- 2 tablespoons of dried burnet leaves
- 1 liter of water

Preparation: Put the dried leaves into a pot with water. Simmer over low heat for about 10 minutes. After this time, strain the infusion.

Great Burnet infusion can be used as a rinse for washing wounds and inflammatory skin conditions. It can also be taken orally to soothe sore throat and mouth.

Great Burnet Mixture for External Use

Ingredients:
- 100 g of dried burnet leaves
- 500 ml of coconut oil

Preparation: Add the dried leaves to the oil in a pot. Heat over low heat for about 2 hours. Strain the mixture through a fine sieve or cheesecloth, then store in a glass jar.

The Great Burnet mixture can be used as an ointment for wounds, burns, and inflammatory skin conditions. Remember to test on a small area of skin before full application to ensure no allergic reaction occurs

Great Burnet Gargle

Ingredients:
- 2 teaspoons of dried burnet leaves
- 1 cup of water

Preparation: Add the dried leaves to the water in a pot. Simmer over low heat for about 10 minutes. Cool down and strain the liquid.

Great Burnet gargle can be used to rinse the throat in case of sore throat, inflammations, ulcers, or post-operative conditions.

Great Burnet, though little known, is an extremely valuable plant in the world of natural medicine. It has been used for centuries in the treatment of many ailments, particularly due to its strong hemostatic and anti-inflammatory properties.

This means that Great Burnet is a valuable resource for people suffering from various skin conditions such as eczema, acne, or ulcers.

Its strong anti-inflammatory action makes it effective in alleviating irritation and redness, speeding up the healing process.

Great Burnet contains unique compounds such as flavonoids and polyphenols, which contribute to its healing action.

These natural ingredients work synergistically, helping to minimize bleeding, reduce inflammation, and promote healing.

In the era of conventional medicine, despite the growing reliance on pharmaceuticals, plants like Great Burnet still play a crucial role.

Used in the form of ointments, rinses, or compresses, Great Burnet is a natural, effective way to improve skin health.

It is a reminder of the powers of nature that are still relevant, even in our modern world.

The use of plants such as Great Burnet in our daily routine can be a powerful complement to modern healthcare, showing that nature and science can go hand in hand for our health and wellbeing.

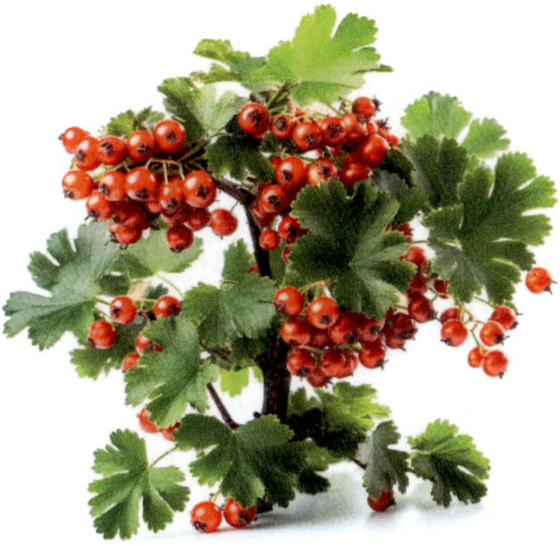

Hawthorn (Crataegus monogyna)
Hawthorn is commonly used to improve heart function, lower blood pressure, and alleviate symptoms of heart failure.

Hawthorn flower infusion

Ingredients:
- 2 teaspoons of dried hawthorn flowers
- 1 cup of water

Preparation: Add the dried hawthorn flowers into a cup. Pour boiling water over the flowers and let it sit covered for about 15 minutes. Strain the infusion.

Hawthorn flower infusion can be used to support heart function, lower blood pressure, alleviate symptoms of heart failure, as well as relieve stress and insomnia.

Hawthorn Fruit Tincture

Ingredients:

- 200 g fresh hawthorn fruits
- 1 litr of alcohol (e.g., vodka)

Preparation: Wash and dry the hawthorn fruits, then place them in a large jar. Pour the alcohol over the fruits, making sure they are completely covered. Seal the jar tightly and store it in a dark place for about 3-4 weeks. After this time, strain the tincture through a tightly woven cloth to separate the fruits from the liquid.

Hawthorn fruit tincture can be used to support heart function, lower blood pressure, and alleviate symptoms of heart failure.

Hawthorn Fruit Jam

Ingredients:

- 1 kg hawthorn fruits
- 1 kg sugar
- Juice from 1 lemon

Preparation: Wash the hawthorn fruits and remove the stems. Transfer the fruits to a large pot, add enough water to cover them, and simmer on low heat until softened. Strain the cooked fruits through a sieve, collecting the juice. Add the sugar and lemon juice to the juice and simmer on low heat, stirring until the sugar is dissolved. Continue cooking the jam until it thickens, then transfer it to sterilized jars.

Hawthorn fruit jam can be used as a healthy addition to bread, pastries, and desserts. It has many health benefits, including supporting heart function.

Hawthorn Flower Syrup

Ingredients:
- 2 cups of hawthorn flowers
- 1 liter of water
- 1 kg of sugar

Preparation: Wash the hawthorn flowers and place them in a large pot. Pour water over the flowers and simmer on low heat for about 30 minutes. Strain the infusion through a sieve, collecting the liquid. Add sugar to the liquid and continue cooking on low heat, stirring until the sugar dissolves. Cook the syrup until it thickens, then transfer it to sterilized bottles.

Hawthorn flower syrup is a delicious and healthy addition to tea, desserts, or cocktails. It can help improve heart function, lower blood pressure, and alleviate symptoms of heart failure.

Hawthorn Leaf Infusion

Ingredients:
- 1 teaspoon of dried hawthorn leaves
- 1 cup of boiling water

Preparation: Pour boiling water over the hawthorn leaves and let it steep covered for about 10 minutes. Strain the infusion and sweeten with honey or sugar if desired.

Hawthorn leaf infusion helps to alleviate symptoms of stress and heart failure. It can be used as a natural calming remedy.

Flavonoids: Hawthorn is rich in flavonoids, which have strong antioxidant properties. They help fight free radicals in the body, contributing to protection against various diseases, including heart diseases.

Oligomeric proanthocyanidins (OPCs): These are plant compounds belonging to the flavonoid group, and they possess strong antioxidant and anti-inflammatory properties..

Vitamins and Minerals: Hawthorn contains vitamins such as vitamin C and some B vitamins, as well as minerals like potassium, magnesium, and calcium.

Organic Acids: Hawthorn also contains organic acids, such as citric acid and malic acid.

Proteins and Fats: Hawthorn contains small amounts of proteins and fats, which are important for overall health.

Hawthorn, scientifically known as Crataegus monogyna, is a plant species that has been used in natural medicine for centuries. Its unique properties make it an invaluable resource for the heart and cardiovascular system.

For many cultures, hawthorn symbolizes the heart and is considered the „heart herb." This symbolism is not only metaphorical but also reflects the actual health benefits that hawthorn can provide to our cardiovascular system.

With the presence of various bioactive compounds such as flavonoids and proanthocyanidins, hawthorn acts as a natural beta-blocker, helping to control blood pressure and heart rhythm.

It also acts as an adaptogen, assisting the body in coping with stress. Stress, both physical and emotional, is a significant risk factor for many heart diseases, so hawthorn's ability to alleviate the effects of stress is immensely valuable. Moreover, hawthorn may help combat certain menopausal symptoms such as hot flashes and insomnia. This versatility makes it a versatile and universal plant in natural healthcare.

Discovering the power of plants like hawthorn reminds us that medicine doesn't always have to rely on complicated technologies and expensive drugs. Sometimes, the answers to our most pressing health issues may lie in the simplicity and potency of nature.

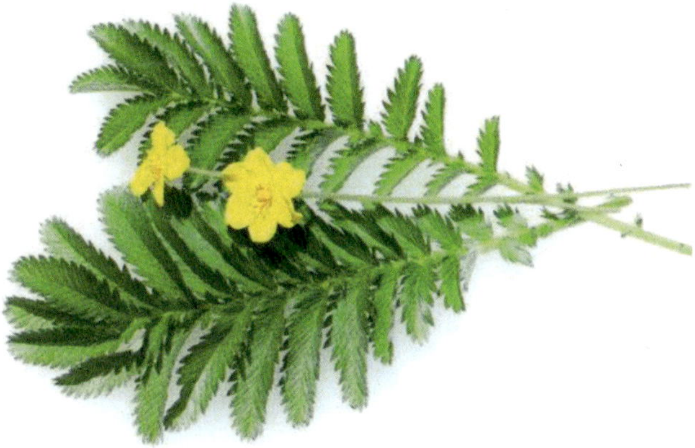

Silverweed (Potentilla anserina)
Silverweed has antidiarrheal and anti-inflammatory properties, and it is often used to treat diarrhea and inflammatory conditions of the gastrointestinal system.

<u>**Silverweed Tea**</u>

Ingredients:
- 1-2 teaspoons of dried silverweed leaves
- 1 cup of boiling water

Preparation: Pour boiling water over the silverweed leaves and steep for about 10 minutes. After this time, the tea should be ready to drink. You can drink it 2-3 times a day, especially in case of digestive issues.

Silverweed tea can help alleviate digestive problems such as diarrhea and inflammatory conditions of the gastrointestinal system.

Silverweed Tincture

Ingredients:
- 200 g dried silverweed leaves
- 1 liter of vodka

Preparation: Place the silverweed leaves in a large jar and pour vodka over them. Seal the jar tightly and store it in a dark and cool place for about 2 weeks. After this time, strain the tincture and transfer it to a bottle.

Silverweed tincture can be used to treat inflammatory conditions and digestive issues. You can take 1-2 teaspoons of the tincture 2-3 times a day.

Silverweed Throat Pain Potion

Ingredients:
- 2 tablespoons of dried silverweed leaves
- 1 cup of water
- 1 tablespoon of honey

Preparation: Pour boiling water over the dried leaves and let them steep for about 15 minutes. After this time, strain the infusion and add a tablespoon of honey to it.

You can drink this potion 2-3 times a day in case of throat pain.

Silverweed has anti-inflammatory properties that can help alleviate throat pain. The addition of honey not only enhances the taste of the potion but also adds additional healing properties.

Silverweed Face Mask

Ingredients:
- 1 tablespoon of dried silverweed leaves
- 2 tablespoons of plain yogurt

Preparation: Grind the dried silverweed leaves into a fine powder. Then, mix it with the yogurt until you achieve a smooth consistency. Apply the mask to your face and leave it on for about 15 minutes, then rinse off with warm water.

Silverweed has anti-inflammatory properties that can help treat skin inflammations. The yogurt, on the other hand, moisturizes and nourishes the skin, making the mask ideal for skincare.

Silverweed Compote

Ingredients:

- 1 of fresh silverweed leaves
- 1 liter of water 1/2 cup of sugar (or to taste)

Preparation: Wash the silverweed leaves and add them to a pot with water. Cook over low heat for about 15-20 minutes. Then, add sugar and cook for an additional 5 minutes until the sugar is completely dissolved. Strain the compote through a sieve and let it cool.

Silverweed compote is a delicious and healthy beverage that can be enjoyed both hot and cold. Silverweed has anti-inflammatory properties, which can be beneficial for the digestive system.

Silverweed Leaf Salad

Ingredients:

- A handful of fresh silverweed leaves
- 1 tomato
- 1 cucumber, olive oil
- Salt and pepper to taste

Preparation: Wash the silverweed leaves and pat them dry. Chop the tomato and cucumber into bite-sized pieces. In a salad bowl, combine the silverweed leaves, tomato, and cucumber. Drizzle with olive oil and season with salt and pepper to taste. Toss everything together until well combined.

Silverweed leaf salad is a refreshing and nutritious dish.

The silverweed leaves add a unique flavor and texture to the salad, while the tomato, cucumber, and olive oil provide additional freshness and taste.

Flavonoids: These are potent antioxidants that can help combat free radicals in the body. They may also aid in the prevention of certain types of cancer.

Tannins: These compounds have astringent and anti-inflammatory properties. They can assist in the treatment of inflammatory conditions of the digestive system, such as diarrhea.

Vitamins and Minerals: Silverweed contains small amounts of vitamins and minerals, such as vitamin C and potassium. Vitamin C is important for immune function and collagen production, while potassium is essential for the proper functioning of the heart and muscles.

Ellagic Acid: This organic acid is a well-known antioxidant that has potential anticancer properties.

Remember to ensure that the plant is healthy and grows in a clean environment, away from pollutants such as traffic, agricultural chemicals, and other toxins.

We gather herbs following the principles of sustainable harvesting, avoiding the destruction of entire plant populations and always leaving a portion of the plants untouched so that they can continue to grow and reproduce.

Each plant we gather is a valuable source of life that deserves our respect and care. Without proper harvesting and nurturing, we may lose these valuable resources that are so important for our health and well-being.

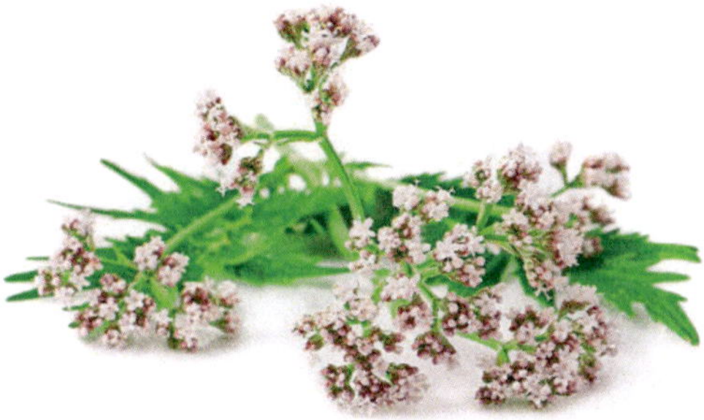

Valerian (Valeriana officinalis)
Valerian is commonly used for the treatment of insomnia and anxiety due to its calming properties.

Valerian, also known as Valeriana officinalis, is a remarkable plant that has been a valuable component of natural medicine for centuries. Originating from Europe and Asia, valerian has gained a reputation for its nerve-soothing powers and is often referred to as„nature's tranquilizer" due to its potent calming properties and aid in combating insomnia.

What makes valerian so special is its unique combination of active ingredients that naturally interact with our nervous system. Valerenic acids, bioactive compounds present in the plant, have the ability to increase the levels of gamma-aminobutyric acid (GABA) available in the brain - a neurotransmitter that promotes relaxation and helps reduce anxiety.

Valerian Infusion

Ingredients:
- 1 tablespoon of dried valerian root
- 1 cup of boiling water

Preparation: Pour boiling water over the valerian root and let it steep for 10 minutes. Strain and drink the infusion before sleep. This will help in treating insomnia and anxiety.

Valerian Tincture

Ingredients:
- 100 g of valerian root
- 500 ml of alcohol (40-60% content)

Preparation: Pour the alcohol over the valerian root and let it sit for about 2 weeks, shaking the contents every few days. After this time, strain and store in a dark, cool place.

Use by adding a few drops to a glass of water or tea before sleep to support sleep and alleviate anxiety.

Valerian Herbal Blend

Ingredients:
- 2 parts valerian
- 1 part lemon balm
- 1 part hops

Preparation: Combine the herbs and pour boiling water over them, let it steep for about 10 minutes. Strain and drink before sleep.

This blend is ideal for individuals suffering from insomnia and nervo-usness, as all three herbs have calming properties.

Valerian Essential Oil

Ingredients:
- Dried valerian root
- Grape seed oil

Preparation: Fill a jar halfway with dried valerian root, then pour grape seed oil over it, completely covering the herb. Close the jar and let it sit in a dark, cool place for about 6 weeks, shaking the contents every few days. After this time, strain the oil and store it in a dark bottle.

You can use it for massage, which can help alleviate stress and tension.

Alkaloids: Valerian contains alkaloids that can affect the nervous system and contribute to its calming effects.

Valepotriates: These compounds are one of the key components of valerian and have strong calming and anti-anxiety properties.

Valerenic acid and isovaleric acid: These acids have calming and relaxing effects.

Flavonoids: These components are potent antioxidants that can help protect the body from the harmful effects of free radicals.

Minerals: Valerian contains minerals such as potassium, calcium, and magnesium, which are essential for proper bodily function.

Vitamins: Although valerian is not particularly rich in vitamins, it contains small amounts of B vitamins, which are important for the health of the nervous system.
The power of valerian extends beyond treating insomnia and anxiety. This plant is also valued for its antispasmodic abilities, making it a valuable tool in alleviating menstrual pain, muscle cramps, and similar conditions.

In the context of our stressful, always-on-the-go lifestyle, providing our mind and body with affordable, natural, and effective support is a valuable advantage. And as demonstrated by the herb known as valerian, nature is incredibly capable of providing us with such solutions.

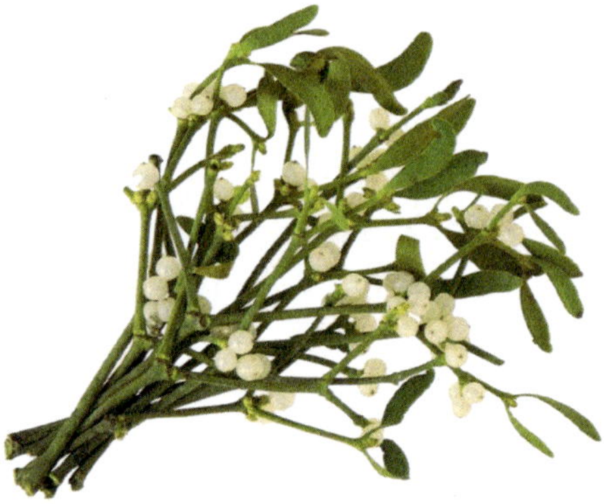

Mistletoe (Viscum album)

White mistletoe is used in the treatment of hypertension and improving heart function, but it is also being investigated for its potential use in cancer treatment. Mistletoe, also known as Viscum album, is an extraordinary plant that has consistently captivated the attention of both botanists and naturopathic physicians for centuries. Known for suspending itself at heights, mistletoe possesses a unique ability to survive by growing on various species of trees and drawing essential nutrients from them. However, what makes mistletoe particularly special in the context of natural medicine is its numerous potential health benefits.

The medicinal properties of mistletoe are attributed to its complex profile of active ingredients, including numerous alkaloids, lectins, polysaccharides, amino acids, and flavonoids. Among them are substances that exhibit blood pressure-lowering, calming, and heart-strengthening effects. These components make mistletoe a valuable tool in the prevention and treatment of cardiovascular diseases such as hypertension. However, the benefits of mistletoe extend beyond supporting heart health.

Mistletoe, also known as Viscum album, is an extraordinary plant that has consistently captivated the attention of both botanists and naturopathic physicians for centuries. Known for suspending itself at heights, mistletoe possesses a unique ability to survive by growing on various species of trees and drawing essential nutrients from them. However, what makes mistletoe particularly special in the context of natural medicine is its numerous potential health benefits.

The medicinal properties of mistletoe are attributed to its complex profile of active ingredients, including numerous alkaloids, lectins, polysaccharides, amino acids, and flavonoids. Among them are substances that exhibit blood pressure-lowering, calming, and heart-strengthening effects. These components make mistletoe a valuable tool in the prevention and treatment of cardiovascular diseases such as hypertension. However, the properties of mistletoe do not end with supporting heart health.

White Mistletoe Infusion

Ingredients:

- 1 teaspoon of dried white mistletoe
- 1 cup of boiling water

Preparation: Place the dried mistletoe in a cup. Pour boiling water over it and let it steep for approximately 10 minutes. Strain the infusion and drink it.

White mistletoe infusion is used in traditional medicine to alleviate the symptoms of hypertension.

Tincture of White Mistletoe

Ingredients:
- 100 g dried white mistletoe
- 500 ml vodka

Preparation: Place the dried white mistletoe in a jar. Pour vodka over it, then tightly seal the jar. Store it in a dark place for 2-3 weeks, shaking the jar daily. After this time, strain the tincture through a sieve or coffee filter into another container.

White Mistletoe Oil

Ingredients:
- 1 cup of dried white mistletoe
- 1 liter of olive oil

Preparation: Place the dried white mistletoe in a jar. Pour olive oil over it. Seal the jar tightly. Store it in a dark, cool place for 4-6 weeks. Strain it through a coffee filter or sieve into another container.

White mistletoe oil can be used externally for massaging painful areas or to improve circulation. The properties of mistletoe may support the health of blood vessels and the heart.

Note: It is important to remember that this is for external use only, and white mistletoe oil should not be consumed. The use of mistletoe, both internally and externally, should be done under the supervision of a specialist. White mistletoe tincture is used in traditional medicine to improve heart function and lower blood pressure.

White mistletoe contains numerous potentially toxic compounds, such as lectins and alkaloids, which can have various negative effects on the body, including nausea, vomiting, and even damage to the heart or liver. All of this makes white mistletoe a plant with high toxic potential.

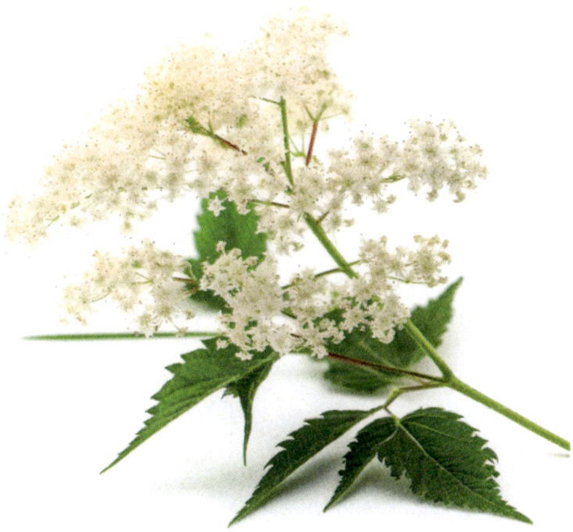

Meadowsweet (Filipendula ulmaria)
Meadowsweet has analgesic and anti-inflammatory properties, often used in the treatment of joint inflammations.

<u>Meadowsweet Infusion</u>

Ingredients:
- 1 tablespoon of dried meadowsweet
- 1 cup of boiling water

Preparation: Add 1 tablespoon of dried meadowsweet to a cup or container. Pour boiling water over the herb. Cover the container and let it steep for about 15 minutes. After that time, strain the infusion into another cup, discarding the herbs.

Meadowsweet infusion has analgesic and anti-inflammatory effects, making it suitable for relieving pain and inflammation, especially related to the musculoskeletal system. Drink 1-2 cups of the infusion daily, preferably in the morning and evening.

Compress with Meadowsweet

Ingredients:
- Handful of fresh meadowsweet leaves
- Gauze or clean cloth

Preparation: Gather fresh meadowsweet leaves and wash them under running water. Crush the leaves into a paste, you can use a mortar and pestle. Apply the paste onto a clean cloth or gauze.

A meadowsweet compress has analgesic and anti-inflammatory effects. It can be applied to painful joints or areas with inflammation. Keep the compress on the skin for about 15-20 minutes, several times a day.

Meadowsweet Tincture

Ingredients:
- 100g dried meadowsweet
- 500ml alcohol (such as diluted 40-60% ethanol or vodka)

Preparation: Place 100g of dried meadowsweet in a clean, dry jar. Pour alcohol over the herbs, filling the jar completely and ensuring they are fully covered. Seal the jar and store it in a dark, cool place for 2 weeks, shaking it daily. After two weeks, strain the tincture through cheesecloth into a clean bottle, squeezing out as much liquid as possible.

Meadowsweet tincture has analgesic and anti-inflammatory effects.

It can be taken orally, diluted in a glass of water, 10-15 drops 2-3 times a day, particularly for joint pain and rheumatism.

It can also be used externally by applying it topically to the affected areas.

Meadowsweet Syrup

Ingredients:
- 2 cups of fresh meadowsweet flowers
- 4 cups of sugar

Preparation: Place fresh meadowsweet flowers in a glass jar and cover them with sugar. Cover the jar and leave it in a warm place for 2-3 days until the sugar completely dissolves and forms a syrup. Stir occasionally to expedite the process. Once the sugar is dissolved, strain the syrup into a clean jar through a fine sieve or cheesecloth.

Meadowsweet syrup is a natural analgesic and anti-inflammatory remedy. It can be used internally, such as adding 1-2 teaspoons to tea or hot water 2-3 times a day.

It can also be used externally, for example, for rinsing wounds.

Meadowsweet has a somewhat distinctive appearance, but it is possible to confuse it with other species from the rose family, especially with other Filipendula species.

For example, young meadowsweet plants may be mistaken for young plants of the palmate meadowsweet (Filipendula palmata). Both of these plants have similar, finely divided leaves. However, palmate meadowsweet leaves are usually darker and more shiny, and its flowers are pink, not white like those of meadowsweet.

Another species that can be confused with meadowsweet is dropwort (Filipendula vulgaris). These two plants have similar leaves and flowers, but dropwort is usually shorter and has smaller flowers.

Flavonoids: Meadowsweet contains numerous flavonoids, which are compounds with confirmed anti-inflammatory and antioxidant effects.

Salicylates: Meadowsweet is rich in salicylic compounds, which are natural sources of salicylates. These compounds have anti-inflammatory and analgesic properties, which is why they are often used in the treatment of joint inflammations and pain.

Triterpenes: Meadowsweet also contains triterpenes, which exhibit a range of beneficial biological properties, such as anti-inflammatory, antibacterial, and antifungal effects.

Tannins: Meadowsweet contains tannins, which have astringent properties. Therefore, they are often used in the treatment of diarrhea and gastrointestinal issues.

Ellagic Acid: Ellagic acid is a powerful antioxidant that has potential anticancer effects.

To summarize, meadowsweet is truly a gem of nature. It holds valuable treasures in the form of various beneficial components for our health, including vitamins, minerals, and particularly salicylates, which are natural compounds with anti-inflammatory and analgesic properties.

However, meadowsweet should not be used in chronic rheumatologic conditions. Both the leaves and flowers of meadowsweet have been used in folk medicine for centuries. They are used to alleviate both internal and external pain.

Infusions and decoctions from this plant are excellent remedies for headaches, muscle and joint pain, as well as stomach discomfort.

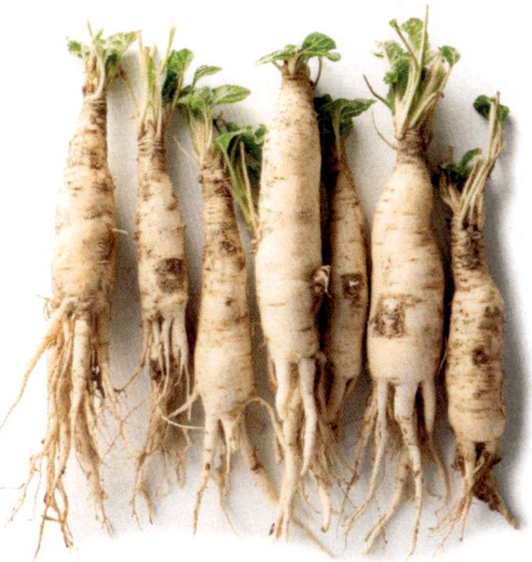

Horseradish Root (Armoracia rusticana)
Horseradish root, also known as horseradish, has traditionally been used for treating respiratory infections and as an appetite stimulant

Horseradish Root Juice

Ingredients:
- Horseradish root
- Lemon (optional)

Preparation: Clean and peel the horseradish root. Crush or grate it, and then squeeze out the juice. If desired, you can add lemon juice for flavor.

Horseradish root juice can be used as a homemade remedy for respiratory infections. It can be consumed once a day, but keep in mind that it is very potent, so always dilute it with water.

Pain-relieving Horseradish Root Compress

Ingredients:
- Horseradish root

Preparation: Clean and peel the horseradish root. Grate it. A horseradish compress has pain-relieving properties.

It can be applied to painful areas, such as joints. However, remember not to leave it on the skin for too long, as it may cause irritation.

Horseradish Root Paste

Ingredients:
- 1 horseradish root
- 1/4 cup of apple cider vinegar
- Salt to taste

Preparation: Peel and thoroughly wash the horseradish root. Grate it using a fine grater. Add apple cider vinegar and salt to taste, mix well. Transfer the paste to a jar and seal it tightly. Store in the refrigerator.

Horseradish root paste, also known as grated horseradish, is a traditional condiment used in many dishes, especially meats and sausages. Apart from its flavor, horseradish is known for its health benefits, including appetite stimulation and digestion support.

Vitamins: Horseradish is rich in vitamins, particularly vitamin C, which is a potent antioxidant. It also contains small amounts of B vitamins, including B1 (thiamine), B2 (riboflavin), B3 (niacin), B5 (pantothenic acid), B6 (pyridoxine), and B9 (folate)..

Minerals: Horseradish provides various minerals such as potassium, calcium, magnesium, phosphorus, as well as trace amounts of iron, copper, zinc, and manganese.

Plant Compounds: Horseradish contains various plant compounds, including glucosinolates, which are natural components found in cruciferous vegetables and are believed to be responsible for many health benefits of horseradish. These glucosinolates transform into isothiocyanates when the plant is cut or grated, giving horseradish its characteristic sharp taste.

Fiber: Horseradish is also a source of fiber, which is beneficial for the health of the digestive system.

Horseradish is a plant that has deep roots not only in the soil but also in the long history of natural medicine. While for many people, horseradish is primarily associated as a condiment, its root holds much more potential than meets the eye. On one hand, horseradish root is a true treasure trove of bioactive ingredients. It is rich in vitamin C, potassium, calcium, magnesium, phosphorus, as well as phytoncides, which exhibit strong antibacterial properties. Additionally, it contains glucosinolates, sulfur compounds that give horseradish its characteristic pungent aroma and taste.

Glucosinolates are also active components attributed to the antiviral, antibacterial, and antifungal properties of horseradish. However, a broader perspective on the use of horseradish emerges when viewed through the lens of natural medicine. Traditionally, horseradish root has been utilized as a warming remedy, stimulating circulation and supporting the immune system. Its strong, pungent nature also has the ability to stimulate appetite and aid digestion. However, horseradish root also has its place in modern phytotherapy.

Due to its strong antibacterial and antiviral properties, it is sometimes used as a supportive treatment for upper respiratory tract infections. Furthermore, studies suggest that the components found in horseradish may have anticancer effects.

In summary, horseradish root is undoubtedly worth exploring. Its uses in the kitchen and natural medicine are just the beginning of discovering its full potential. And most importantly, horseradish is an excellent example of how nature offers us ingredients that can support our health on various levels. It is worth buying horseradish from organic farmers and then experiencing and enjoying its potential and wonderful taste.

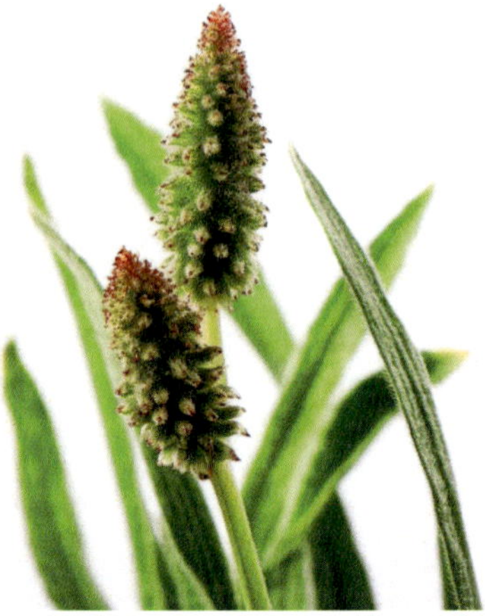

Ribwort Plantain (Plantago lanceolata)
Common Plantain is used as a soothing remedy for cough, as an anti--inflammatory agent, and to accelerate wound healing.

Syrup from Ribwort Plantain for Cough

Ingredients:
- 2 full cups of fresh Ribwort plantain leaves
- 1 cup of sugar or honey
- 1 cup of water

Preparation: Wash and dry the Ribwort plantain leaves. In a saucepan, place the leaves, add water, and simmer over low heat for about 10 minutes. After that, strain the leaves, and return the remaining infusion to the saucepan. Add sugar or honey and continue cooking for about 15 minutes. Once cooled, transfer the syrup to a bottle.

Ribwort plantain syrup helps to soothe cough and throat inflammation. Take one tablespoon of the syrup three times a day.

Compress of Ribwort Plantain for Wounds

Ingredients:
- Several leaves of ribwort plantain

Preparation: Wash the ribwort plantain leaves, pat them dry, and crush them into a paste.

A compress made from ribwort plantain helps to speed up wound healing and reduce inflammation. Apply it to the wound for 15-20 minutes, several times a day.

Remember to always gather plants from locations away from roads and pollutants.

Ribwort Plantain Tea

Ingredients:
- 2 teaspoons of dried ribwort plantain leaves
- 1 cup of boiling water

Preparation: Pour boiling water over the dried ribwort plantain leaves. Leave the infusion covered for about 10 minutes, then strain it.

Ribwort plantain tea helps to soothe cough, sore throat, and inflammation of mucous membranes. You can drink it 2-3 times a day.

Throat Rinse Mixture

Ingredients:
- 1 tablespoon of dried leaves of ribwort plantain
- 1 cup of boiling water

Preparation: Pour a tablespoon of dried ribwort plantain leaves with boiling water. Wait for 10 minutes, then strain it. Gargle with ribwort plantain rinse 2-3 times a day. This can help with sore throat, cough, and prevent the development of infections.

Ribwort Plantain Ointment for Wound Healing

Ingredients:

- 1 cup of dried ribwort plantain leaves
- 1 cup of coconut oil
- 1/4 cup of beeswax

Preparationie: Pour the coconut oil over the dried ribwort plantain leaves and heat on low heat for about 2 hours, stirring occasionally. Strain the mixture through a fine sieve or cheesecloth, squeezing out as much oil as possible. Add the beeswax to the warm oil and stir until the wax completely dissolves. Transfer the finished ointment to a sterile glass jar and let it cool.

Ribwort plantain ointment helps to accelerate wound healing and reduce skin inflammation. Apply a thin layer of the ointment to the wound and cover it with a bandage. Clean the wound and change the bandage at least once a day.

Always remember that any deep or infected wound should be shown to a doctor

Vitamins: Ribwort plantain contains vitamins from the B group (especially B1, B2, B3, and B6), which support the functioning of the nervous system and metabolism. It also contains vitamin C, which has antioxidant properties, supports the immune system, and is necessary for collagen production.

Minerals: This plant is a source of many essential minerals, including calcium (supports bone and teeth health), magnesium (important for muscle and nerve function), potassium (regulates blood pressure), and iron (necessary for hemoglobin production).

Phenolic Acids: Ribwort plantain contains phenolic acids that have strong antioxidant and anti-inflammatory properties. They can help protect the body against damage caused by free radicals and inflammation.

Mucopolysaccharides: Ribwort plantain is known for its content of mucopolysaccharides, which have soothing and protective effects on mucous membranes.

Iridoids: Ribwort plantain contains iridoids (such as aucubin), which have strong antibacterial and anti-inflammatory properties.

Ribwort plantain, also known as Plantago lanceolata, is one of those humble and often underestimated gifts of nature that hold unexpected richness. Although for many people, it is nothing more than a plant that grows practically everywhere - in lawns, by roadsides, in parks - for enthusiasts of natural medicine, ribwort plantain is a true gem.

This plant, also known as the „noble healer," stands out for its remarkable health properties. It possesses outstanding antibacterial, anti-inflammatory, and astringent abilities, making it an invaluable ally in the fight against various infections and inflammatory conditions.

Ribwort plantain plays a special role in treating respiratory ailments. Its leaves are rich in substances called mucopolysaccharides, which have the ability to secrete mucus. This natural „mucus" helps soothe irritated mucous membranes, which is particularly useful for coughs, colds, or asthma.

But that's not the end of ribwort plantain's capabilities. Its leaves, rich in nutrients such as beta-carotene, calcium, vitamin C, and K, can be consumed raw by adding them to salads or smoothies. It also has beneficial effects on the digestive system, alleviating stomach pain, indigestion, and constipation.

Ribwort plantain is also highly valued as an ingredient in natural cosmetics. Its soothing and regenerative properties make it often used in the treatment of minor wounds, burns, insect bites, and skin inflammations such as eczema. In summary, ribwort plantain is a plant whose potential deserves recognition. Its versatile applications and easy accessibility make it one of the most practical and universal ingredients in natural medicine. The plant has been utilized in folk medicine for hundreds, if not thousands, of years. Its health benefits were known in ancient times, where it was used as an anti-inflammatory, antibacterial agent, and for wound healing. Ancient civilizations such as the Romans and Greeks made use of its medicinal properties, and it also enjoyed popularity in traditional Eastern medicine, such as Ayurveda and Chinese medicine.

❖

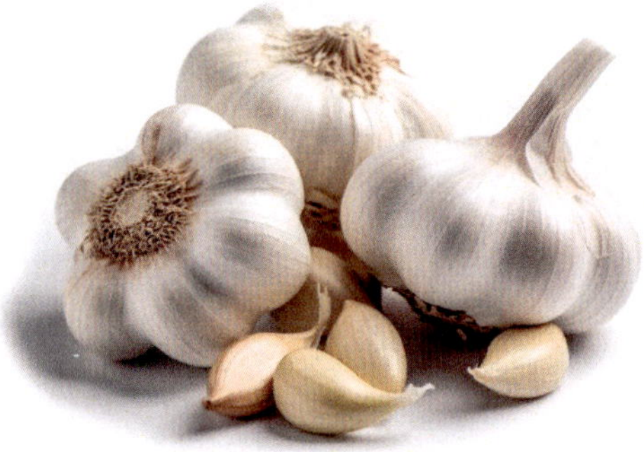

Garlic (Allium sativum)
Garlic has strong antibacterial, antiviral, and antifungal properties. It supports the immune system and improves overall body condition.

<u>Raw Garlic for Boosting the Immune System</u>

Ingredients:
- 1-2 cloves of garlic

You can consume the chopped garlic cloves directly or add them to dishes such as salads, sauces, or soups

Garlic Syrup

Ingredients:

- 8 cloves of garlic
- 1 cup of honey or sugar

Preparation: Crush the garlic and mix it with honey or sugar. Let it sit for 24 hours, then strain it.

Garlic syrup is an excellent homemade remedy for colds and flu. Take 1 teaspoon three times a day.

Garlic Honey

Ingredients:

- 3 heads of garlic
- 500 g of honey

Preparation: Peel the garlic and press it through a garlic press. Mix the garlic with honey and let it sit in a dark place for 3 days.

Garlic honey strengthens the immune system. Consume 1 tablespoon daily.

Garlic Oil

Ingredients:

- 1 garlic bulb
- 2 cups of olive oil

Preparation: Peel and chop the garlic cloves and place them in a jar. Pour olive oil over the garlic and seal the jar. Store it in a dark, cool place for 2 weeks, then strain it.

Garlic oil is great for cooking but also serves as a natural antibacterial remedy for external use. It can be used to moisturize the skin for various skin issues.

Garlic and Lemon Drink

Ingredients:

- 2 cloves of garlic
- Juice of 1 lemon
- 1 cup of warm water

Preparation: Crush the garlic and mix it with lemon juice. Add warm water and stir well.

Garlic and lemon drink is excellent for flu and colds. Drink it 1-3 times a day.

Garlic and Honey for Flu

Ingredients:

- 1 clove of garlic
- 1tablespoon of honey

Preparation: Chop the garlic into small pieces and mix it with honey.

The garlic and honey mixture has antibacterial and antiviral properties. Consume 1 tablespoon of the mixture 2-3 times a day.

Garlic and Ginger Tea

Ingredients:

- 1 clove of garlic
- Small piece of fresh ginger
- 1 cup of water

Preparation: Chop the garlic and ginger into small pieces. Pour boiling water over them and let it steep for 10 minutes.

Garlic and ginger tea helps in fighting flu and colds. Drink it 2-3 times a day

Vitamins: Vitamin C: Known for its role in supporting the immune system and collagen production. B vitamins, including B1 (thiamine), B6 (pyridoxine), as well as small amounts of other B vitamins. B vitamins have multiple functions, including supporting energy production in the body and aiding in the function of the nervous system.

Selenium: Important for thyroid health and the immune system.

Manganese: Important component of many enzymes in the body.

Iron: Essential for red blood cell production.

Calcium: Important for bone and teeth health.

Phosphorus: Supports the maintenance of healthy bones and teeth.

Allicin: A sulfur compound that gives garlic its characteristic odor and taste. Allicin is also responsible for many of garlic's health benefits, such as its antibacterial, antiviral, and antifungal properties.

Flavonoids: Natural plant compounds that exhibit strong antioxidant activity, protecting the body's cells from damage.

Sulfur compounds: Garlic contains various sulfur compounds that may have beneficial effects on health, such as anti-inflammatory properties, heart and blood vessel protection.

Garlic, this commonly known culinary ingredient, is actually a valuable ally to our health and a treasure trove of powerful forces that have roots in both traditional medicine and esoteric beliefs. The power of garlic, appreciated for centuries, combines practical, spiritual, and scientific aspects, creating a fascinating blend that transcends time and cultures. As a dietary ingredient, garlic is rich in sulfur compounds, such as allicin, which exhibit strong antibacterial and antifungal properties.

In ancient Scandinavian, Germanic, and Slavic societies, garlic was an invaluable tool in combating diseases, helping to maintain health and strengthen immunity in times when modern medicine was not available. Modern science confirms these ancient practices, recognizing garlic as a natural antibiotic and one of the most potent allies of the immune system. Garlic's power is also attributed to its significance in esotericism. Many ancient cultures, from the Vikings to the Slavs, attributed to garlic the power to ward off evil spirits and negative energy. Thus, garlic was not only a medicine but also a protective talisman, a symbol of purification and safeguarding.

This spiritual role of garlic is still present in many traditions and rituals, and its presence at the threshold of a home or hanging above the doors is a universal symbol of protection.

In the field of pharmacy, garlic holds significant importance as well. The components of garlic are currently being investigated for their potential in treating various conditions, from heart diseases to cancer. Many scientists appreciate garlic for its polyphenols, antioxidants, and phytosterols, which can help combat inflammatory and oxidative processes in the body.

Garlic, this humble yet powerful gift of nature, is evidence that the deepest wisdom lies in the simplest things. Its universal application, both in terms of health and spirituality, makes it a true treasure of natural medicine, pharmacy, and esotericism, demonstrating how closely intertwined these three aspects of our existence are.

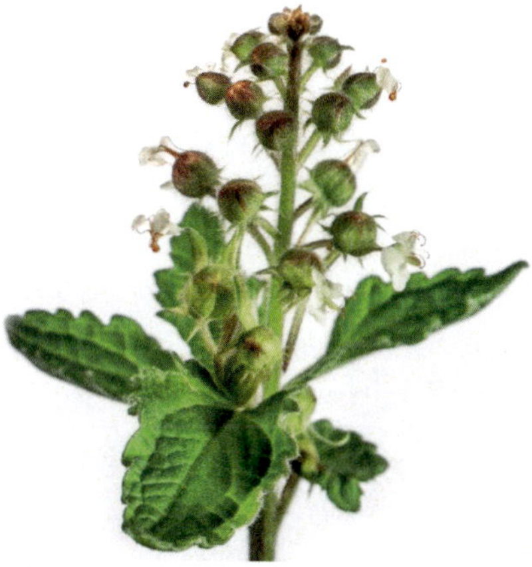

Knotted Figwort (Scrophularia nodosa)
Knotted Figwort, has been used as an antibacterial, anti-inflammatory, and laxative remedy. It is highly valued for its properties by many tribes around the world.

Knotted Figwort Infusion

Ingredients:
- 2 tablespoons of dried knotted figwort leaves
- 1 cup of boiling water

Preparation: Pour boiling water over the knotted figwort leaves and let it steep for about 15 minutes. Strain and allow it to cool.

Knotted figwort infusion has antibacterial and anti-inflammatory properties. It can be consumed 2-3 times a day for a better sense of well-being, especially during colds and infections.

Knotted Figwort Ointment

Ingredients:
- Handful of dried knotted figwort leaves
- 1 cup of coconut oil

Preparation: In a small saucepan, heat the coconut oil until completely melted. Add the dried knotted figwort leaves and simmer on low heat for about 30 minutes. After that time, strain the mixture and pour it into a tightly sealable jar. Store in a cool place.

Knotted figwort ointment has anti-inflammatory and antibacterial properties. It can be used topically on the skin to treat minor infections, wounds, and burns.

Knotted Figwort Tonic

Ingredients:
- 1 tablespoon of dried knotted figwort leaves
- 1 liter of water
- 1 tablespoon of honey (optional)

Preparation: Add the knotted figwort leaves to a pot of water and simmer on low heat for 30 minutes. After that time, strain the tonic and add honey for taste if desired. Allow it to cool.

Knotted figwort tonic helps in detoxifying the body. It can be consumed daily, especially after heavy meals, to improve digestion.

Knotted Figwort Compress

Ingredients:
- Handful of fresh knotted figwort leaves
- Warm water (a small amount)

Preparation: Crush the knotted figwort leaves and add a small amount of warm water to create a paste.

Knotted figwort compress helps accelerate wound healing and reduce inflammation. Apply it to the skin for about 15 minutes, then rinse with warm water. It can be used several times a day.

Knotted Figwort Tincture

Ingredients:
- 100 g of dried knotted figwort leaves
- 500 ml of vodka or grain alcohol
- 1-liter jar

Preparation: Fill the jar with dried knotted figwort leaves, then pour vodka or grain alcohol over them, ensuring that all the leaves are submerged. Close the jar and place it in a dark, cool place for about 2 weeks. After that time, strain the tincture and transfer it to a bottle.

Knotted figwort tincture can be used topically for various skin issues such as acne or minor wounds. Apply about 5-10 drops to the affected area.

Exercise caution with oral consumption, as in some cases, it may be harmful.

Iridoids: This group of organic compounds exhibits anti-inflammatory and antibacterial properties.

Flavonoids: Plant compounds that demonstrate strong antioxidant, anticancer, antiviral, and antiallergic effects.

Phenolic glycosides: They possess antibacterial, anti-inflammatory, and antiviral properties.

Triterpenes: They exhibit anti-inflammatory and anticancer activities

Mineral Ingredients: Such as calcium, magnesium, and potassium, which are essential for proper body functioning.

Knotted figwort, also known as Trędownik, is a medicinal plant with a long history of use in folk medicine, especially in Europe. Its ability to alleviate inflammation, antibacterial action, and laxative properties make it highly valued in herbal medicine.

When it comes to medicinal plants, many of them possess remarkable power due to the rich active compounds they contain. However, some stand out for their accessibility and ease of cultivation, making them even more appealing. Plants containing iridoids, flavonoids, phenolic glycosides, and triterpenes are true treasure troves of natural compounds that can have a significant impact on our health. These substances, which serve as biologically active components in many plants, are responsible for a range of beneficial health effects, including antioxidant, anti-inflammatory, antiviral, antibacterial, and immune-supportive actions. For example, iridoids exhibit potent antibacterial and antifungal activity and can support nervous system health.

Flavonoids are well-known antioxidants that can help combat free radicals and protect against heart diseases. Phenolic glycosides, on the other hand, are valued for their anticancer properties, while triterpenes can have a positive impact on the immune and hormonal systems.

Furthermore, the fact that these plants are readily available and relatively easy to cultivate makes them an ideal choice for those seeking to harness the benefits of nature without compromising on convenience.

Cultivating such plants not only provides a steady supply of fresh, unprocessed ingredients but also offers a delightful way to connect with nature and literally „plant health" in our own gardens.

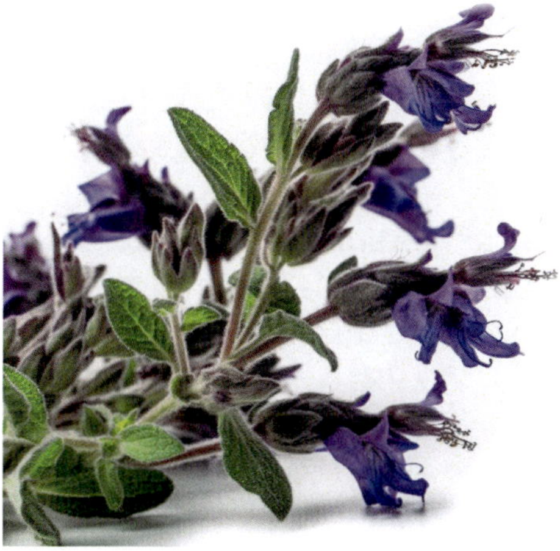

Sage Meadow (Salvia pratensis)
Sage is widely used to improve the function of the digestive system and has strong antiseptic properties.

Meadow Sage Leaf Infusion

Ingredients:
- 2 tablespoons of dried meadow sage leaves
- 1 cup of boiling water

Preparation: Pour boiling water over the sage leaves and infuse, cove-red, for about 10 minutes. Then strain.

The meadow sage leaf infusion has a calming effect on the digestive system, helps with stomach ailments, and acts as an antiseptic. Drink 1-3 times a day.

Meadow Sage Poultice

Ingredients:
- A handful of fresh meadow sage leaves
- A gauze pad or clean cloth

Preparation: Crush the fresh meadow sage leaves until they become a pulp. Then spread it on a gauze pad or clean cloth.

A meadow sage poultice has antiseptic properties. Apply to the area that requires disinfection or acceleration of the wound healing process. Repeat the procedure 1-2 times a day.

Meadow Sage Oil

Ingredients:
- A handful of dried meadow sage leaves
- 1 cup of coconut oil

Preparation: Pour the coconut oil over the sage leaves and put them in a jar, which is then sealed. Leave in a dark, cool place for 2-3 weeks, shaking the jar every few days. After this time, strain the oil and store it in a tightly closed jar.

Meadow sage oil has antiseptic properties and soothes the skin. It can be used externally on the skin for minor inflammatory conditions, irritations, or abrasions.

Meadow Sage Incense

Ingredients:
- Dried meadow sage leaves

Preparation: Roll the dried meadow sage leaves into tight, thick bundles and tie with a string, leave to dry completely.

Bundles of meadow sage can be used as incense for space cleansing. Burning sage releases aromatic smokes that are considered purifying and soothing.

Meadow Sage Cream

Ingredients:

- 1 cup of dried meadow sage leaves
- 1/2 cup of coconut oil
- 1/4 cup of beeswax
- A few drops of sage essential oil (optional)

Preparation: Heat the coconut oil in a saucepan, then add the dried sage leaves to it. Reduce the heat and simmer for about 30 minutes, stirring occasionally. After this time, add the beeswax and stir until it is completely dissolved. Finally, add a few drops of essential oil and stir. Pour the liquid into a container and leave to cool.

Meadow sage cream has antibacterial and antiseptic properties. It can be applied to the skin, especially in the case of minor inflammatory conditions, irritations, or abrasions.

Meadow Sage Ointment

Ingredients:

- 2 cups of fresh meadow sage leaves
- 1 cup of coconut oil
- 1/4 cup of beeswax

Preparation: Wash the sage leaves and dry them with a paper towel. In a small pot, over low heat, melt the coconut oil. Add the sage leaves to the pot and simmer over low heat for about 1 hour, stirring occasionally. After an hour, strain the mixture through a gauze into a clean jar, removing the leaves. Return the pot to the heat and add the beeswax to the oil. Cook over low heat, stirring, until the wax is completely melted. Pour the hot ointment into clean jars or ointment cans. Leave to cool and harden.

Meadow Sage Ointment has antibacterial and anti-inflammatory properties. It can be used for minor cuts, scrapes, burns, skin rashes, and inflammatory skin conditions.

Essential oils: Essential oils in sage, such as thujone, camphor, cineole, have antiseptic, anti-inflammatory, and antibacterial properties.

Flavonoids: Flavonoids are potent antioxidants that help fight free radicals in the body. They help protect cells from damage and can counteract some chronic diseases.

Phenolic acids: Such as rosmarinic acid and caffeic acid, which have anti-inflammatory, antiviral, and antibacterial activity.

Triterpenes: Triterpenes, such as ursolic acid and oleanolic acid, have anti-inflammatory and anticancer activity.

Vitamins and minerals: Meadow sage is also a source of some vitamins, such as vitamin C and B vitamins, and minerals such as potassium, calcium, magnesium, copper, and zinc.

Meadow sage, also known as Norwegian sage, is a wonderful example of a natural remedy used by the ancient Norwegians, including their shamans. This versatile plant, with its strong antiseptic, anti-inflammatory, and medicinal properties, was an essential ingredient in ancient Norwegian healing rituals and medical practices. Sage leaves were used to treat a wide range of ailments - from digestive problems to skin infections. Shamans used this plant not only as a medicine but also as a tool for cleansing spaces and people.

The use of sage oil helped in warding off negative energy, while simultaneously supporting healing processes. These practices stemmed from a deep awareness that the health of the body and mind is inextricably linked with energy balance and harmony with nature.

For the ancient Norwegians, meadow sage was not only an effective medicine, but also a tool enabling a deeper connection with the natural world.

Today, despite technological and medical advances, meadow sage still plays an important role in natural medicine. Its versatile use is proof of the power of nature in treating various ailments.

Moreover, understanding and appreciating the role of sage in both a physical and spiritual context can remind us of the importance of maintaining harmony with nature for our health and well-being.

Meadow sage, with its rich history and versatile applications, remains an important source of inspiration for those seeking natural methods of improving health and well-being, regardless of their cultural context or beliefs.

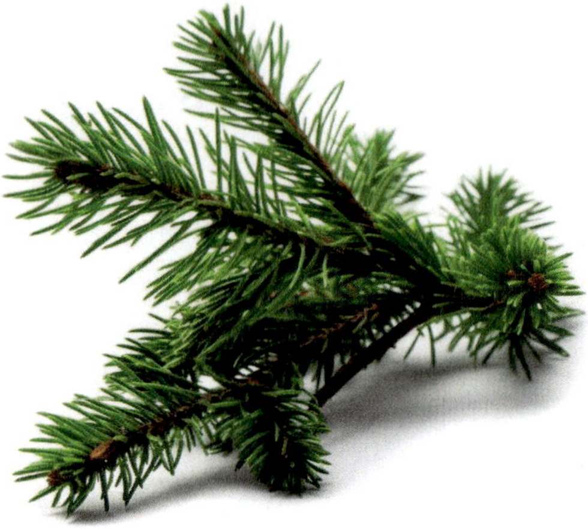

Norway Spruce (Picea abies)
Spruce needles are a rich source of vitamin C, have antiviral and antibacterial effects. They are traditionally used in treating upper respiratory tract infections, soothe coughs and support the immune system. In addition, due to their analgesic properties, they were used for external treatment of muscle and joint pains.

<u>Spruce Needle Infusion</u>

Ingredients:
- 1 A handful of fresh spruce needles
- 1 1 liter of water

Preparation: Rinse the spruce needles under running water, then pour a liter of boiling water over them. Allow it to steep for about 20 minutes, then strain.

The infusion from spruce needles is a rich source of vitamin C and has a strengthening effect on the immune system. It can be used as an addition to tea or drunk independently. Drink 1-2 times a day, especially during the flu season.

Spruce Needle Syrup

Ingredients:
- 1 cup of fresh spruce needles
- 1 cup of sugar
- 1 cup of water

Preparation: Rinse the needles, then throw them into a pot. Add sugar and water, simmer over low heat until the sugar dissolves. Then reduce the heat and cook for about 30 minutes. Strain through a sieve lined with gauze.

Spruce needle syrup is a natural remedy for coughs and respiratory problems. It can be added to tea, drinks or desserts. Store in the refrigerator.

Spruce Needle Oil

Ingredients:
- 2 cups of fresh spruce needles
- 1 cup of oil (e.g., olive oil, coconut oil)

Preparation: Rinse the needles, dry them and pour oil over them in a jar. Seal tightly and set aside for 2 weeks in a dark, cool place. After this time, strain the oil through a sieve lined with gauze.

Spruce needle oil has antiseptic, anti-inflammatory, and analgesic effects. It can be used for massage (e.g., for muscle pain), for baths or as an addition to cosmetics.

Spruce Needle Gargle Mixture

Ingredients:
- 1 tablespoon of dried spruce needles
- 1 cup of boiling water

Preparation: Collect spruce needles. Remember to do this away from pollution and busy roads. Dry the needles, then place a spoonful of needles in a cup or jug. Pour hot, but not boiling water over the needles. Leave the jug covered for about 20 minutes. After this time, strain the mixture into another container. You can use a sieve or gauze for this.

Use the mixture for gargling 2-3 times a day. It will help soothe cold symptoms, sore throat and acts as an antiseptic. Gargling with this mixture can also provide relief in case of inflammatory conditions of the oral cavity.

Spruce Olive Oil

Ingredients:
- Fresh spruce needles
- Olive oil

Preparation: Collect fresh spruce needles, preferably early in the morning when they are the most juicy. Wash them thoroughly, then dry. Then place the needles in a jar, trying to fill its entire capacity. The needles should be loosely packed, not squeezed. Pour clean olive oil over the needles, so they are completely covered. Screw the jar and set it aside in a dark, cool place for about 4-6 weeks. Remember to shake the jar daily. After this time, strain the oil into a clean jar. You can use gauze or a sieve for this.

You can apply spruce olive oil on the skin for massage. It has a soothing effect on the muscles, helps in skin regeneration and has an antiseptic effect. You can also add it to the bath - a few drops of oil dissolved in a bathtub with warm water will bring relief to tired muscles.

Spruce needle compresses

Ingredients:
- A handful of spruce needles
- Gauze or clean cloth
- Hot water

Preparation: Place spruce needles in a container, pour hot water over them and cover. Leave it for about 10 minutes. After this time, soak a gauze or clean cloth in this infusion, squeezing out excess water.

Such prepared compress can be applied to joints or other parts of the body that are sore or tense. Spruce has anti-inflammatory and analgesic properties, and a warm compress can further help relax muscles.

Vitamins and minerals: Spruce needles are a source of vitamins, such as vitamin C, which is important for the immune system. They also contain some minerals such as potassium and calcium.

Terpenes: Terpenes are organic compounds that have strong antioxidant and anti-inflammatory properties. The terpenes found in spruce include α-Pinene and Limonene.

Flavonoids: Flavonoids are antioxidants that can protect the body from free radicals and have anti-inflammatory effects.

Tannins: Tannins are compounds that have strong antibacterial and anti-inflammatory effects. They can also speed up wound healing.

Resins: The resins contained in spruce needles have anti-inflammatory, analgesic and antibacterial properties.

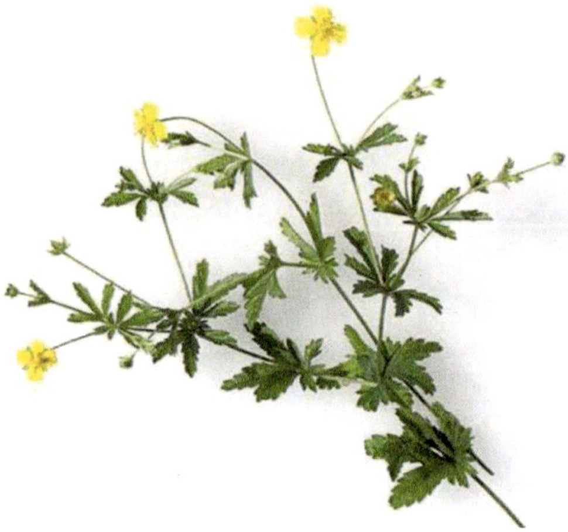

Silverweed (Potentilla anserina)
This plant is known for its anti-diarrheal, anti-inflammatory, and astringent properties. It is traditionally used to treat indigestion and digestive system issues, as well as a soothing remedy for throat irritations. Externally, it can be used to treat minor cuts and wounds, thanks to its properties that accelerate healing.

Silverweed infusion

Ingredients:
- 2 tablespoons of dried silverweed
- 1 cup of boiling water

Preparation: Pour 1 cup of boiling water over 2 tablespoons of dried silverweed and leave it to infuse for about 10 minutes. Then, strain the infusion.

The silverweed infusion can be used to alleviate indigestion and digestive system problems. Drink it twice a day, in the morning and in the evening.

This plant is known for its anti-diarrheal, anti-inflammatory, and astringent properties. Traditionally, it is used to treat indigestion and digestive issues, as well as to soothe throat irritations. Topically, it can be applied to heal minor cuts and scrapes, due to its wound-healing properties.

Silverweed Infusion

Ingredients:
- 2 tablespoons of dried silverweed
- 1 cup of boiling water

Preparation: Pour a cup of boiling water over 2 tablespoons of dried silverweed and let it steep for about 10 minutes. Then strain the infusion.

The silverweed infusion can be used to alleviate indigestion and digestive system issues. Drink it twice a day, morning and evening.

Silverweed Poultice

Ingredients:
- A handful of fresh silverweed leaves
- Gauze or a clean cloth

Preparation: Crush the fresh silverweed leaves into a pulpy mass. Then spread the mass on a gauze or a clean cloth.

A silverweed poultice has analgesic and anti-inflammatory effects. Apply it to the affected areas for 15-20 minutes, several times a day.

Silverweed Gargle

Ingredients:
- 1 tablespoon of dried silverweed
- 1 cup of boiling water

Preparation: Pour a cup of boiling water over a tablespoon of dried silverweed. Leave it to steep for about 10 minutes, then strain it.

A silverweed gargle can be used to soothe throat irritations. Gargle 2-3 times a day.

Vitamin C: This vitamin is a strong antioxidant that supports the immune system, aids in fighting free radicals, and promotes skin health.

Quercetin: This is a type of flavonoid that acts as a potent antioxidant. Quercetin has anti-inflammatory, antiallergic properties, and may help combat infections.

Tannins: Tannins are a group of polyphenols that have antibacterial, anti-inflammatory, antiviral, and antioxidant properties.

Triterpenes: These compounds have antiviral, anti-inflammatory, and anticancer effects.

Flavonoids: Flavonoids are powerful antioxidants that help fight free radicals in the body, preventing cell damage.

Silverweed, also known as potentilla anserina, played a fundamental role in traditional medicine of Scandinavia and tribal cultures of Europe.

This plant is rich in nutrients such as vitamin C, quercetin, tannins, triterpenes, and flavonoids, making it valued for its medicinal properties for centuries. Distinguished by its multitude of uses, silverweed was not only used to treat wounds and alleviate inflammation but also to improve the function of the digestive system. Its roots, rich in tannins, were used to soothe the symptoms of diarrhea and stomach ailments due to their strong astringent and anti-inflammatory properties.

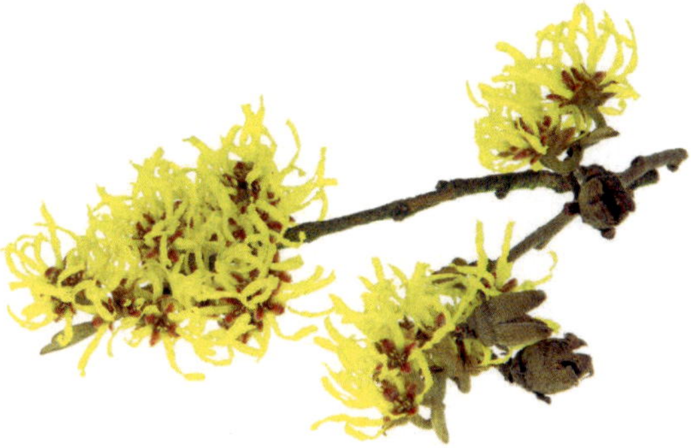

Witch Hazel, known as Hamamelis virginiana (Hamamelis virginiana)
This plant is known for its anti-inflammatory, antibacterial, and antifungal properties. Traditionally, it is used to soothe skin irritations, such as bruises, burns, skin cracks, and also to treat hemorrhoids and skin infections.

Juice from Sedum telephium

Ingredients:
- A handful of fresh sedum leaves.

Preparation: Wash and dry the fresh Sedum telephium leaves. Put the leaves in a juicer and extract the juice.

You can consume Sedum telephium juice once a day to aid its analgesic and anti-inflammatory effects.

Compresses with Carpathian sedum.

Ingredients:

- A handful of fresh sedum leaves.

Preparation: Wash the leaves, dry and crush them thoroughly to release the juices. Then apply it to the sore spot on the skin, cover with a bandage or thick cloth and leave it on for several hours. A poultice from Sedum telephium can be used on burns, ulcers, and to alleviate pain.

Sedum telephium Tea

Ingredients:

- 1 teaspoon of dried Sedum telephium leaves
- 1 cup of boiling water

Preparation: Pour boiling water over the dried Sedum telephium leaves and steep it under a cover for about 10 minutes. After this time, the tea should be ready to drink.

Sedum telephium tea is known for its analgesic and anti-inflammatory properties.

Witch Hazel Face Mist

Ingredients:

- 1/2 cup of witch hazel water
- 1/2 cup of rose water
- A bottle with a spray pump

Preparation: Mix the witch hazel water with the rose water. Then pour the mixture into a bottle with a spray pump.

Spray your face with the mist 2-3 times a day to hydrate the skin and refresh its appearance.

Homemade Facial Tonic

Ingredients:
- 1 cup of witch hazel water
- 1/2 cup of aloe vera
- 1/4 cup of apple cider vinegar
- A few drops of essential oil (e.g., lavender, mint)

Preparation: Combine all ingredients in a small container, mix well.

Apply the tonic to cleansed skin with a cotton pad, avoiding the eye area. Do not rinse. Can be used twice a day.

Honey and Witch Hazel Face Mask

Ingredients:
- 1 tablespoon of honey
- 1 teaspoon of witch hazel water
- 1 teaspoon of coconut oil

Preparation: Mix all the ingredients to get a uniform mass.

Apply the mask to cleansed face skin, avoiding the eye area. Leave it on for 15-20 minutes, then rinse with warm water. Use once a week for the best results.

Tannins: These are polyphenols with strong anti-inflammatory and astringent properties. Tannins are responsible for most of the medicinal properties of witch hazel, including its antibacterial and anti-inflammatory action.

Flavonoids: These are plant compounds with strong antioxidant activity. They can help protect the skin from the harmful effects of free radicals.

Saponins: These are compounds naturally found in many plants that have antibacterial, antifungal, and anti-inflammatory properties.

Gallic Acid: This is an organic compound present in many plants, which has strong anti-inflammatory and antibacterial properties.

Catechins: These are compounds belonging to the group of polyphenols, which show strong antibacterial and anti-inflammatory effects.

Eugenol: This is a chemical compound with strong antibacterial, antiviral, and antiparasitic action.

Safrole: This is an organic compound with anti-inflammatory, antibacterial, and antiviral effects.

Witch hazel, also known as Hamamelis virginiana, is a plant rich in health-beneficial ingredients, such as tannins, flavonoids, and saponins, which have made it a basis for many natural treatments for centuries.

Modern natural medicine, like in the past, values it for its exceptional anti-inflammatory, antibacterial, and antifungal properties. The diversity of applications of witch hazel makes this plant an important element of a natural medicine cabinet.

Tonics and fluids are prepared based on the distillate from leaves and branches, which effectively soothe skin irritations, such as bruises, burns, or cracks. However, the possibilities of using this plant in natural medicine do not end there.

Due to its astringent action, witch hazel is also helpful in treating ailments such as hemorrhoids or various types of skin infections.

But the role of witch hazel in ancient cultures went beyond strictly medicinal use. This plant, due to its strong energy and ability to adapt to various conditions, was often used in esoteric practices.

It was believed to have the power of energetic purification, hence it was used to create various talismans or amulets to protect against negative energy. In the 21st century, despite the continuous development of medicine, witch hazel is still a valuable ingredient in natural healing. Its wealth of active ingredients and wide application make it deserve a place in every home medicine cabinet.

Collect only mature twigs: The best time to harvest witch hazel is late autumn or winter when the plant is fully mature. Then it contains the most active ingredients. Only collect twigs that are healthy and show no signs of disease or pests.

Be mindful of the ecosystem: Witch hazel is an important element of its ecosystem. When collecting, pay attention not to disturb the balance - do not collect all twigs from one plant, always leave some for wildlife and other plants.

Use sharp tools: Use sharp tools when cutting twigs to minimize plant damage.

Remember, too large, careless cuts can lead to infection or damage to the plant.

Collect with respect: Always remember that you are a guest in nature.

Collect with respect for the plants and the environment they are in.

In this way, you will contribute to preserving biodiversity and the health of our planet.

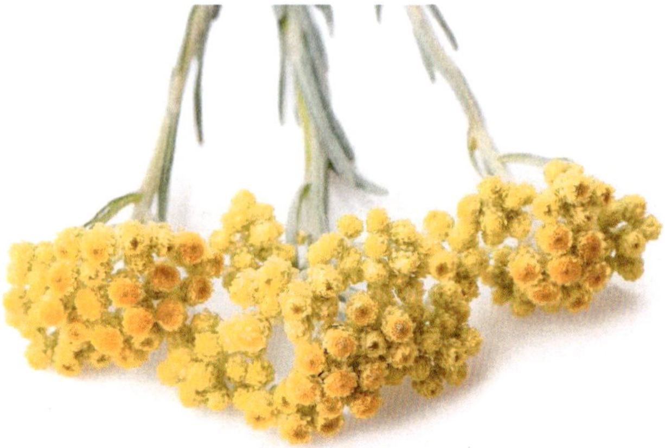

Sandy Everlasting (Helichrysum arenarium)
This plant is valued for its strong anti-inflammatory and antioxidant properties, as well as its support for liver function and digestion. It is also used in the treatment of various skin conditions, such as eczema or burns.

<u>Tea from Sandy Everlasting</u>

Ingredients:
- 1 teaspoon of dried sandy everlasting
- 1 cup of hot water

Preparation: Pour hot water over the dried everlasting. Allow to brew for 10-15 minutes. Strain and allow it to cool a bit before consumption.

You can drink Sandy Everlasting tea 1-2 times a day to support digestion and liver function. It can also be applied externally to the skin to soothe inflammation and accelerate healing.

Sandy Everlasting Oil

Ingredients:
- 1 cup of dried sandy everlasting
- 1 cup of coconut oil or another carrier oil

Preparation: Place the dried everlasting in a jar and cover with oil. Close the jar and shake it a few times to thoroughly mix the ingredients. Leave in a dark, cool place for 2-3 weeks. After this time, strain the oil through a dense sieve or cloth to separate the plant.

Sandy Everlasting oil can be applied externally to the skin to soothe inflammation, heal wounds and burns, and act as a natural antioxidant.

Recipe for a Sandy Everlasting face mask

Ingredients:
- 2 tablespoons of dried sandy everlasting
- 3 tablespoons of plain yogurt
- 1 teaspoon of honey

Preparation: Grind the dried sandy everlasting into a fine powder using a coffee grinder or blender. In a bowl, combine the powder with yogurt and honey. Mix all the ingredients thoroughly to achieve a uniform consistency.

Apply the sandy everlasting mask to cleansed facial skin, avoiding the eye area. Leave on for 15-20 minutes, then rinse with warm water. Using such a mask once a week will help soothe skin inflammation, speed up the healing of minor wounds, and have a nourishing effect.

Sandy Everlasting Bath Infusion

Ingredients:
- 1 cup of dried sandy everlasting
- 2 liters of water

Preparation: Add the dried everlasting and water to a pot. Boil over medium heat for about 15-20 minutes. Allow to cool, then strain.

Add the sandy everlasting infusion to your bath. This will allow you to benefit from the anti-inflammatory properties of the everlasting, as well as help to relax the body after a hard day. It is advisable to spend about 15-20 minutes in such a bath.

However, remember to rinse your skin thoroughly after the bath to avoid irritation.

Sandy Everlasting Lip Balm

Ingredients:
- 2 tablespoons of dried sandy everlasting
- 3 tablespoons of coconut oil
- 1 tablespoon of beeswax

Preparation: Pour coconut oil over the dried sandy everlasting and leave for a few hours to soak. Then add the beeswax and heat the whole on low heat until the wax melts. Strain the mixture through a dense sieve or gauze, leaving only the liquid. Pour the liquid into small jars or lip balm containers and leave to solidify.

The sandy everlasting lip balm can be applied to the lips in case of dryness, cracked lips, and even herpes. Everlasting has anti-inflammatory and healing effects, which will speed up skin regeneration.

Sandy Everlasting Massage Oil

Ingredients:

- Half a cup of dried sandy everlasting
- A cup of oil, e.g. jojoba or sunflowe

Preparation: Pour the oil over the dried sandy everlasting in a jar and close tightly. Leave in a dark, cool place for 2-3 weeks, stirring daily. After this time, strain the oil through gauze into a clean jar.

Sandy everlasting oil can be used for body massage. It has a relaxing and soothing effect on the skin, and can also help alleviate muscle and joint pain..

Flavonoids: These chemical compounds have a strong antioxidant effect, which helps protect our cells from damage caused by free radicals. Flavonoids can also counteract inflammation.

Coumarins: These substances have antibacterial, antifungal, and antiviral properties. They can assist in the treatment of various infections, and may also act as natural anticoagulants.

Phytosterols: These are substances that can help lower the level of „bad" LDL cholesterol in the body, which may prevent the development of cardiovascular diseases.

Polysaccharides: Polysaccharides can help improve the function of the immune system and can act as probiotics that support a healthy gut flora.

Triterpenes: These compounds have anti-inflammatory properties and can aid in the treatment of skin and mucous membrane inflammation.

Sandy everlasting, commonly found on sand dunes and dry sandy areas throughout Europe, was a key element in traditional Germanic, Saxon, and Viking medicine.

Valued for its versatile medicinal properties, it was used to alleviate various ailments such as liver disease, gastrointestinal failure, and as a remedy for skin inflammation.

Used to produce infusions, ointments, or oils, it was a fundamental element of daily health prevention in the communities of these ancient cultures.

Today's research confirms many of these traditional uses, showcasing a wealth of bioactive ingredients such as flavonoids, coumarins, or phytosterols, which have strong antioxidant and antibacterial effects.

Despite the passage of centuries, sandy everlasting remains a symbol of natural treatment, combining the wisdom of ancestors with scientifically confirmed health benefits.

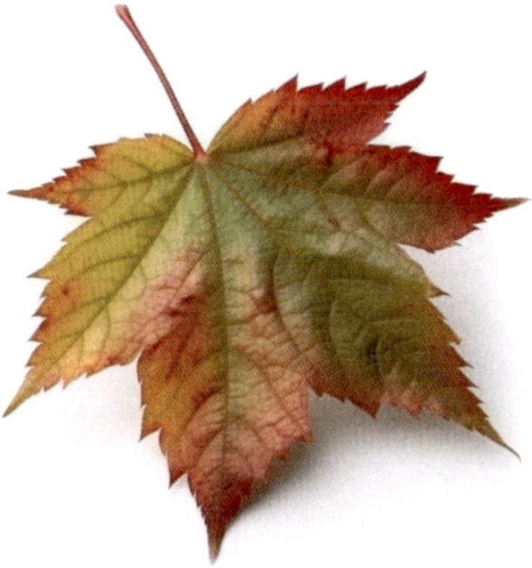

Boxelder Maple (Acer negundo)
This tree is used in traditional medicine for its strong analgesic and antiviral properties. It is also used as an anti-inflammatory agent and in the treatment of respiratory ailments. The hemostatic properties of boxelder maple are used for external treatment of wounds.

Infusion of Boxelder Maple Leaves

Ingredients:
- 1 tablespoon of dried boxelder maple leaves
- 1 cup of boiling water

Preparation: Pour the leaves with boiling water and leave to infuse for about 10 minutes. Strain before consumption.

You can consume it 2-3 times a day to alleviate symptoms of cold and flu, as well as a painkiller.

Ointment with Boxelder Maple Leaves

Ingredients:
- 1 cup of dried boxelder maple leaves
- 1 cup of coconut oil

Preparation: Blend the boxelder leaves with coconut oil. Then, heat the mixture over low heat for about 30 minutes. After this time, strain the mixture and store the ointment in a tightly closed jar.

The ointment can be applied to the skin to alleviate muscle or joint pain, as well as minor cuts and bruises.

Tincture of Boxelder Maple Leaves

Ingredients:
- Half a cup of dried boxelder maple leaves
- 1 cup of 70% alcohol

Preparation: Place the leaves in a jar, pour the alcohol so that the leaves are completely covered. Close the jar and place it in a dark, cool place for about 2-4 weeks, stirring daily. After this time, strain the liquid and store in a dark bottle.

The tincture can be used externally on the skin to alleviate skin irritations, muscle or joint pain. For internal use, consult a doctor.

Compress with Boxelder Maple Leaves

Ingredients:
- A few fresh boxelder maple leaves

Preparation: The leaves should be thoroughly washed, then softened, e.g. with the help of a mallet.

The compress can be applied to the area of pain (e.g. joints, muscles), securing with a bandage. Leave for about 20-30 minutes.

Flavonoids: Flavonoids are a group of plant compounds that have strong antioxidant properties. They may help protect the body from free radicals and cell damage.

Anthocyanins: This group of flavonoids give boxelder maple leaves their autumnal red and purple color. Anthocyanins have antioxidant properties and may have benefits for heart and brain health.

Phenolic acids: Such as ferulic acid, caffeic acid, and chlorogenic acid. They have strong antioxidant and anti-inflammatory properties.

Triterpenes: These compounds have many potential health benefits, including antibacterial, anti-inflammatory, and anticancer properties.

The boxelder maple, also known as Acer negundo, has a long history of use both in natural medicine and in the shamanic practices of ancient cultures. It would undoubtedly have been valued by the ancient Vikings, who were looking for effective and natural ways to treat ailments. Originating from North America, the boxelder maple has strong analgesic and antiviral properties, and its leaves, roots, and bark were used to treat various ailments. For example, a decoction from the leaves could be used to alleviate pain and reduce inflammation, while a root decoction could serve as an anti-cough medicine, alleviating respiratory system ailments.

Ancient shamans could have utilized these properties in their rituals and healing practices, much as they are in today's healing traditions. The essence of these practices was the understanding that the health of body and mind is closely linked to energetic balance and harmony with nature. In today's pharmacology, boxelder maple continues to be appreciated for its medicinal properties.

Scientific research confirms its effectiveness in treating various ailments, and its extracts are often used in the production of medicines. Many pharmaceutical companies are conducting research into new applications for boxelder maple, underlining the ongoing importance of this plant for medicine.

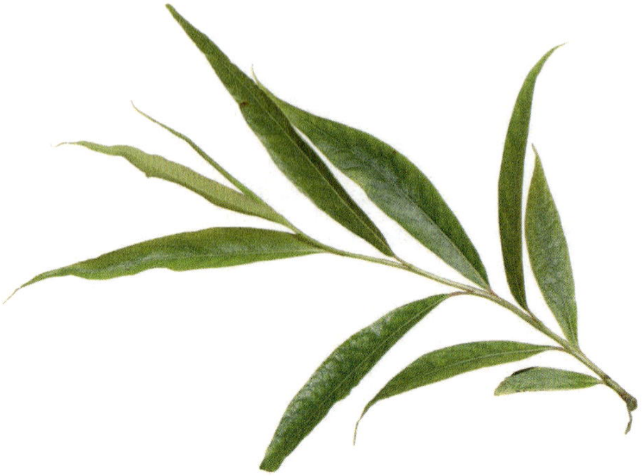

White Willow (Salix alba)
The bark of the white willow is a source of methyl salicylate, a natural form of salicylic acid, from which aspirin is made. It has anti-inflammatory and analgesic properties. The most valued part of this tree is the bark, which contains salicin, a chemical compound with analgesic and antipyretic action, also a precursor to aspirin.

Willow bark infusion

Ingredients:
- 1-2 easpoons of dried white willow bark
- 1 scup of water

Preparation: Pour water into a pot and add the dried willow bark. Bring to a boil and simmer over low heat for about 10-15 minutes. Strain and allow the infusion to cool down.

You can drink the willow bark infusion 2-3 times a day to alleviate headaches, muscle pains, toothaches, or menstrual discomfort.

Willow Bark Macerate

Ingredients:
- 1 part dried white willow bark
- 5 parts alcohol (e.g., vodka)

Preparation: Add dried willow bark to a jar and pour over the alcohol. Close the jar and leave it in a dark, cool place for about 2 weeks. Shake the jar every day. After 2 weeks, strain the macerate through a fine cheesecloth or coffee filter and store in a dark bottle.

The macerate can be applied externally to painful areas on the skin, bruises, or swellings. It can also be used internally, after consultation with a doctor, as an analgesic and anti-inflammatory agent.

Honey with Willow Bark

Ingredients:
- 1 cup of honey
- 1/4 cup of dried white willow bark

Preparation: Add dried willow bark to a jar, then pour over the honey. Close the jar and leave it in a dark, cool place for 2-3 weeks, stirring every few days. After this time, strain the honey and store in a clean jar.

Honey with willow bark can be consumed by the spoonful once a day as a natural analgesic and anti-inflammatory agent.

Willow Bark Compress

Ingredients:

- 1 cup of dried white willow bark
- 2 cups of water

Preparation: Boil water in a pot and add dried willow bark. Simmer over low heat for about 15 minutes. Strain the infusion and wait until it cools down to a skin-acceptable temperature.

Soak a cloth or sponge in the infusion and apply to painful areas, e.g., bruises, swelling, or muscle pain. This can be done 2-3 times a day.

Salicin: This is the main component of willow bark, which in the body converts to salicylic acid, acting as an analgesic and anti-inflammatory.

Flavonoids: These are plant antioxidants that have many health benefits, including protection against heart disease and some types of cancer.

Tannins: They have astringent, antibacterial, and anti-inflammatory properties, making them effective in treating minor wounds and ulcers.

Phenolic acids: They have anti-inflammatory and antibacterial properties.

Triterpeny: They may contribute to lowering cholesterol levels and have anti-inflammatory properties.

White willow (Salix alba), thanks to its extraordinary medicinal properties, deserves special recognition in the context of European and Scandinavian natural medicine.

Valued for its analgesic and anti-inflammatory effects, it has been used by herbalists across the continent for centuries. Methyl salicylate, a natural form of salicylic acid, which is the main ingredient of aspirin, is found in white willow bark. It is due to this component that white willow was traditionally used to alleviate pain and inflammatory conditions.

Apart from its role in folk medicine, white willow also has a long history of use in rituals and religious ceremonies in Scandinavia, where it was considered a sacred tree. Knowledge of traditional plant-based medicine, like white willow, helps us better understand not only our cultural roots but also the potential that lies in nature.

White willow is an excellent example of how humans can utilize the gifts of nature for health and well-being improvements.

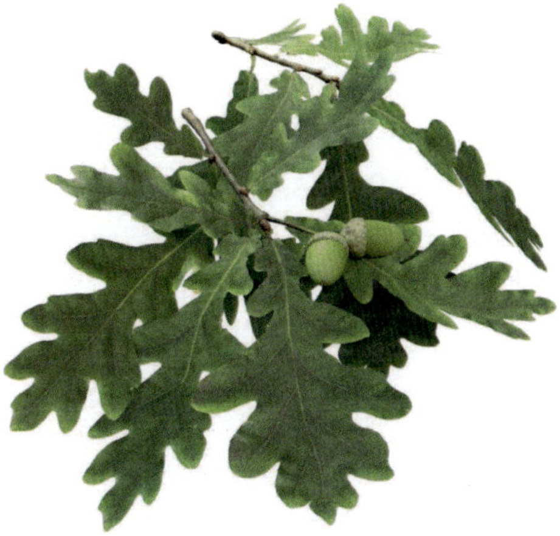

English Oak (Quercus robur)
Oak bark has traditionally been used to treat various ailments, including diarrhea, hemorrhoids, throat inflammation, and skin inflammatory conditions.

Oak Bark Infusion for Throat Rinsing

Ingredients:

- 2 tablespoons of oak bark
- 1 cup of boiling water

Preparation: Pour 2 tablespoons of oak bark with a cup of boiling water. Set aside for 20 minutes to infuse. Strain and gargle 2-3 times a day.

Oak Bark Compress for Hemorrhoids

Ingredients:

- 3 tablespoons of oak bark
- 1 liter of boiling water

Preparation: Pour 3 tablespoons of oak bark with a liter of boiling water. Set aside for 30 minutes to infuse. Strain and leave to cool.

Soak a clean cloth or gauze in the solution and apply to the area affected by hemorrhoids for 15-20 minutes. Repeat 2-3 times a day.

Oak Bark Decoction for Diarrhea

Ingredients:

- 1 tablespoon of oak bark
- 1 cup of water

Preparation: Put a tablespoon of oak bark into a pot with water. Simmer over low heat for about 15 minutes. Strain and let it cool down.

Drink 1/3 cup 3 times a day until the diarrhea subsides.

Oak Bark Face Mask for Acne

Ingredients:
- 1 teaspoon of ground oak bark
- 2 teaspoons of green clay
- Water

Preparation: Combine the ground oak bark and green clay in a small dish. Add enough water to create a smooth paste.

Apply the mask to your face, avoiding the area around the eyes. Leave it on for 10-15 minutes, then rinse with warm water. Apply a moisturizing cream.

Oak Bark Decoction for Ulcers and Wound

Ingredients:
- 1 tablespoon of oak bark
- 1 liter of water

Preparation: Add the oak bark to the water in a pot. Simmer over low heat for about 20 minutes. Let it cool down and strain.

The decoction can be used to rinse wounds and ulcers 2-3 times a day.

Oak Bark Foot Soak for Sore Feet

Ingredients:
- 1/2 cup of oak bark
- 2 liters of water

Preparation: Add the oak bark to a pot of water. Simmer over medium heat for about 20 minutes. Strain and pour into a bowl. When the decoction cools down to a pleasant temperature, immerse your feet in it for 15-20 minutes.

This relaxing soak helps with foot pain and fatigue. It can be used daily.

Gargle with Oak Bark

Ingredients:
- 2 tablespoons of finely chopped oak bark
- 1 liter of water

Preparation: Pour water into a pot, add oak bark. Simmer on low heat for about 20 minutes. Strain the decoction and let it cool down.

Use as a gargle 2-3 times a day, especially in case of sore throat or tonsillitis.

Oak Bark Tea for Diarrhea

Ingredients:
- 1 teaspoon of finely chopped oak bar
- 1 cup of water

Preparation: Pour water into a pot, add oak bark. Simmer on low heat for about 15 minutes. Strain the decoction and let it cool down.

Drink small portions throughout the day to alleviate diarrhea symptoms.

Tannins: The bark of the English oak is particularly rich in tannins, which have astringent, anti-inflammatory, and antibacterial properties. Tannins may help in treating inflammatory skin conditions, diarrhea, and can also alleviate hemorrhoid symptoms.

Flavonoids: These are potent antioxidants that may protect the body from the harmful effects of free radicals.

Triterpenes: They have antibacterial and anti-inflammatory effects, and can also support skin health.

Organic acids: They may help in digestion and improve overall gut health

Minerals: Oak bark also contains various minerals, including calcium, potassium, magnesium, zinc, and iron.

The English oak, a majestic tree with a massive trunk and spreading crown, played a key role in the lives of ancient European cultures such as the Celts, Germans, and Vikings, and its importance in natural medicine is undeniable. The Celts revered the English oak as a sacred tree, considered a symbol of strength, endurance, and longevity. In their culture, the oak was seen as a gateway to other worlds, playing a vital role in spiritual practices.
Druids, the Celtic clergy, often gathered under oaks to conduct their rituals and ceremonies. They are credited with discovering the medicinal properties of oak bark, which they used to treat many ailments, including diarrhea, hemorrhoids, and inflammatory skin conditions. The Vikings and Germans also enjoyed the benefits of the English oak.

They took advantage of its properties in their healing practices, while simultaneously recognizing the oak as a symbol of masculinity and strength, often likening it to their gods, such as Thor and Donar.

In natural medicine, the English oak is valued for its strong astringent, anti-inflammatory, and antibacterial properties. Oak bark, rich in tannins, is used to prepare infusions, decoctions, and ointments that are used to treat various ailments. Ointments made from oak bark can help alleviate inflammatory skin conditions, while infusions and decoctions can help alleviate diarrhea and digestive problems.

In modern times, despite the advances in medicine, the English oak is still valued for its medicinal properties. Extracts from oak bark are used in the production of many pharmaceutical and cosmetic products, confirming the enduring contribution of this powerful tree to human well-being. This tree surrounds us almost everywhere, whether it is in Poland, Germany, Scandinavia or the distant Caucasus, it is a treasure trove of magnificent properties.

Remember them when you need them!

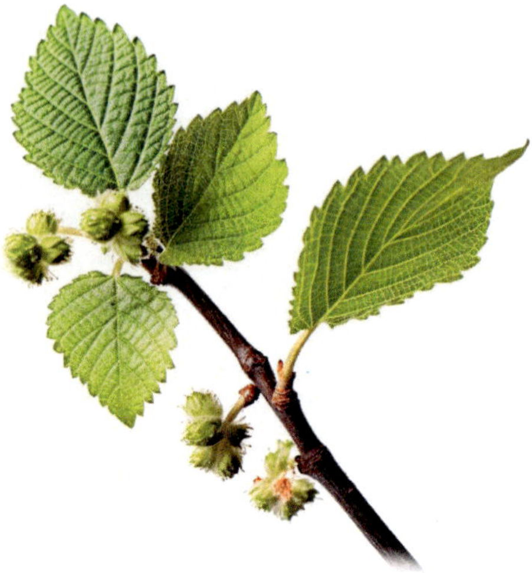

Common Hazel (Corylus avellana)
The hazel is known for its nuts, which are rich in protein, fats, vitamins, and minerals.

Hazelnut Snack

Ingredients:
- Hazelnuts

Preparation: Hazelnuts can be eaten raw as a healthy snack. They are tasty and satisfying, while providing many valuable nutrients.

Hazelnuts can also be added to various dishes - salads, desserts, cakes, or muesli.

They are an excellent source of energy for athletes and people leading an active lifestyle.

Hazelnut Oil

Ingredients:
- Hazelnuts

Preparation: Preparation: Oil can be obtained from hazelnuts, which is a rich source of healthy fats. This is a complex and time-consuming process, so it's easiest to buy ready-made hazelnut oil in the store.

Hazelnut oil can be used both in the kitchen (for salads or baking) and in cosmetics. It moisturizes and nourishes the skin excellently, and is also suitable for hair care.

Infusion of Hazel Leaves

Ingredients:
- Hazel leaves
- Boiling water

Preparation: Pour boiling water over a few hazel leaves and steep covered for about 10 minutes. Strain before consuming.

An infusion of hazel leaves can be used in the treatment of digestive system ailments, such as stomach aches.

Honey from Hazel Flowers

Ingredients:
- Hazel flowers
- Honey

Preparation: Honey can be prepared from freshly collected hazel flowers (best collected in spring). The flowers should be covered with sugar or poured with honey and left for a few weeks in a dark and cool place. After this time, the honey should be strained. Honey from hazel flowers has a delicate, floral taste. It can be added to tea or on sandwiches. It strengthens the body, especially during colds.

Hazel Bark Infusion

Ingredients:
- Hazel bark
- Boiling water

Preparation: Pour a cup of boiling water over 1 tablespoon of finely crushed bark and steep covered for about 15 minutes. Strain before consuming.

Hazel bark infusion has analgesic and anti-inflammatory effects, therefore it can be used for sore throats, oral cavity ailments, and stomach aches.

Compress with Hazel Leaves

Ingredients:
- Hazel leaves

Preparation: Hazel leaves should be poured over with boiling water, wait until they soften, and then wrap in gauze or a bandage. Application: Such a prepared compress can be used for various types of bruises, swellings, or painful joints.

Vitamins: Hazelnuts are an excellent source of vitamin E, which is a potent antioxidant. It helps protect cells from damage caused by free radicals. Additionally, they contain good amounts of B-group vitamins, such as thiamine, riboflavin, niacin, pantothenic acid, pyridoxine, and folates.

Minerals: Hazelnuts are rich in many minerals, including copper, manganese, potassium, calcium, iron, magnesium, zinc, and selenium. Copper and manganese are important for maintaining healthy bones and the production of red blood cells, while magnesium helps in the proper functioning of muscles and nerves.

Protein: Hazelnuts are an excellent source of plant protein, which is necessary for the building and repair of tissues in the body.

Fats: Although hazelnuts are quite calorific, most of the fat they contain is healthy monounsaturated and polyunsaturated fats. They also contain small amounts of omega-3 fatty acids..

Fiber: Hazelnuts are also a good source of fiber, which helps maintain a healthy digestive system and is beneficial for heart health.

The hazel, a characteristic tree and shrub of European forests, has for centuries provided abundant crops of nuts, which were valued for their nutritional and medicinal value. Particularly the Vikings, but also Druids and other ancient communities, knew and appreciated the power carried by this humble nut. For the Vikings, hazelnuts were an important part of the diet. These were protein, fat, and fiber-rich foods that provided necessary energy during the long Scandinavian winters and sea voyages. The Vikings also understood that hazelnuts are a valuable source of many important minerals, such as magnesium, iron, and zinc, which help maintain health and efficient body function.

The Druids, in their deep connection with nature, saw in the hazel not only a source of food but also a tool for ritual and medicinal purposes. Hazelnuts were often used in divination practices, and oil from hazelnuts was used for massage to alleviate muscle and joint pains. The Druids also believed that the hazel has the power to bring wisdom and inspiration, making it a significant element of their spiritual practices. In modern times, natural medicine still uses hazelnuts for various medicinal purposes.

These nuts are known for their antioxidant content, which helps fight free radicals and support overall health conditions. Thanks to the content of vitamin E, hazelnuts are often used in the cosmetic industry to produce creams and oils that moisturize the skin and help fight aging. The hazel and its nuts are evidence of how nature can provide us with valuable resources on many levels: nutritional, medicinal, spiritual, and cosmetic.

This humble plant, appreciated both in antiquity and in contemporary pharmacy, continues its multifaceted action for the health and well-being of people.

❖

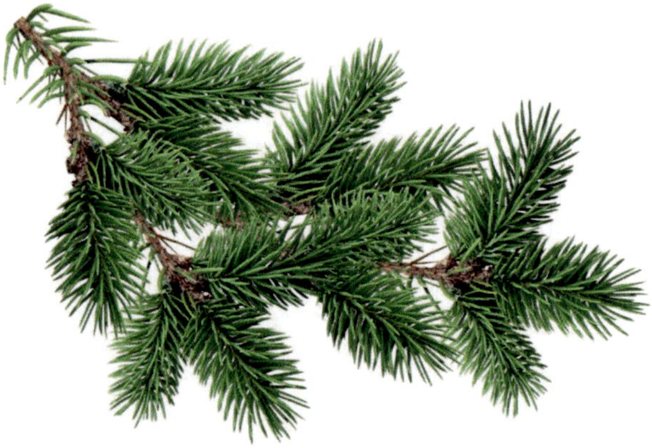

Balsam Fir (Abies balsamea)
Juices and resins from this tree are used as a natural remedy for colds and coughs.

Balsam Fir Cough Syrup

Ingredients:

- 2 cups of fresh balsam fir buds
- 2 cups of sugar
- 1 cup of water

Preparation: Place the fir buds in a jar. In a pot, bring the sugar and water to a boil, stirring until the sugar dissolves. Pour the hot mixture over the buds in the jar. Cover the jar and leave it for 24 hours. The next day, strain the syrup through a fine sieve or cloth. Store the syrup in the refrigerator.

Use 1 tablespoon of the syrup 2-3 times a day for cough and cold.

Balsam Fir Ointment

Ingredients:
- 1 cup of fresh balsam fir resin
- 1/2 cup of coconut oil
- 1/4 cup of beeswax

Preparation: In a pot, melt the balsam fir resin, coconut oil, and beeswax, stirring constantly. When everything is combined, remove from heat and let it cool. Pour the ointment into a small, clean jar.

Apply the ointment to the skin in case of minor wounds, burns, skin rashes, and also for muscle massage for pain.

Balsam Fir Needle Decoction for Immunity Boost

Ingredients:
- 1 cup of fresh balsam fir needles
- 1 liter of water

Preparation: Wash the spruce needles and place them in a saucepan. Add water and bring it to a boil. Simmer on low heat for about 20 minutes. Strain the decoction and let it cool.

Drink 1-2 cups of the decoction daily to boost immunity.

Balsam Fir Massage Oil

Ingredients:
- 1 cup of fresh balsam fir needles and buds
- 2 cups of vegetable oil (e.g., olive oil, grapeseed oil)

Preparation: Wash the needles and buds, dry them, and place them in a jar. Pour over with the vegetable oil and close the jar. Leave in a warm place for about 2 weeks. After this time, strain the oil through a fine sieve or cloth. Store in a dark place.

Use the oil for body massage, especially for muscle and joint pains.

Balsam Fir Bud Cough Syrup

Ingredients:

- 1 cup of fresh balsam fir buds
- 1 cup of sugar
- 1 cup of water

Preparation: Wash and dry the buds, then place them in a pot. Add sugar and water, and bring to a boil. Simmer on low heat for about 30 minutes. Strain the syrup through a fine sieve or cloth and pour into a clean jar.

Take a teaspoon of the syrup 3 times a day for cough.

Relaxing Bath with Balsam Fir Needles

Ingredients:

- 2 cups of fresh balsam fir needlesj
- Bathwater

Preparation: Wash the needles and place them in a linen bag or in linen cloth tied into a pouch. Place the pouch with the needles in the bathtub and fill it with warm water. Leave for 15-20 minutes, to let the needles release their essential oils.

Take a bath, relaxing in the aromatic water for about 15-20 minutes.

Essential Oils: from this plant contain various components such as limonene, alpha-pinene, and beta-pinene, which have antiseptic, anti--inflammatory, and expectorant (aiding the expulsion of mucus from the respiratory tract) effects.

Resin: The resin from balsam fir is rich in terpenes, which act as natural antioxidants.

Vitamin C: The leaves, or needles, of the fir are a rich source of this key vitamin, which is important for the immune system and skin health.

The Balsam Fir, also known as Abies balsamea, is a coniferous tree native to North America, which has also found its place in the Scandinavian landscape and medicine.

Highly valued by ancient Vikings, druids, and other Nordic cultures, this coniferous tree had many health benefits that were invaluable in the harsh conditions of the Scandinavian climate.

Undoubtedly the most valuable part of the tree is its resin, which is rich in antiseptic terpenes and is used to treat many ailments. The Vikings, who were known experts in using the gifts of nature, often collected the resin from the balsam fir to treat wounds, thereby speeding up the healing process and minimizing the risk of infection.

These properties were invaluable in times when antibiotics were still unknown. Additionally, the resin was used to treat respiratory diseases. Inhalations with balsam fir resin were popular among Vikings who suffered from respiratory tract infections. This natural remedy helps in clearing the respiratory tract, relieving cough, and alleviating symptoms of asthma.

In modern times, the balsam fir is still used in natural medicine and aromatherapy. Its strong antiseptic, anti-inflammatory, and disinfecting properties are utilized. Its essential oil is used in skincare products, in wound healing, and also in bath products and massage oils, which help to alleviate stress and tension.

Spirituality and medicine were inseparable for the Vikings, and the balsam fir was often regarded as a sacred tree, which helped in connecting with nature and divinity..

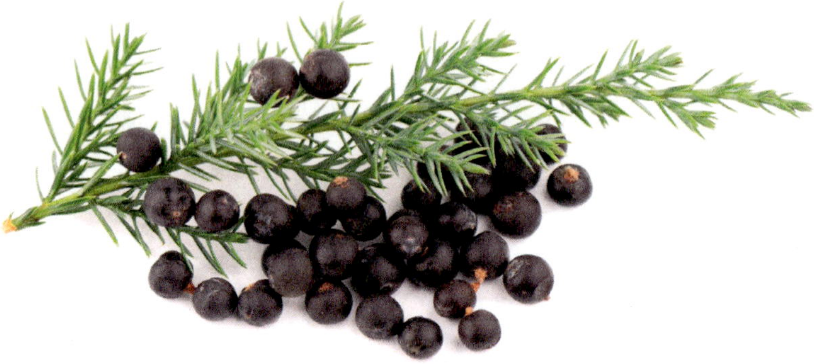

Common Juniper (Juniperus communis)
Juniper berries are used in the treatment of urinary tract infections, digestive problems, and to improve the functioning of the immune system. Below is a picture of already dried juniper fruits, in their fresh form they are purple.

Juniper Berry Infusion

Ingredients:
- 1 teaspoon of dried juniper berries
- 1 cup of hot water

Preparation: Pour hot water over the juniper berries and leave to infuse for about 15 minutes. Strain and drink once a day.

The juniper infusion helps improve digestion and has a diuretic effect. It may help in urinary tract infections.

Juniper Berry Tincture

Ingredients:
- 1 cup of dried juniper berries
- 500 ml of spirits

Preparation: Put the juniper berries in a jar, then pour over the spirits. Leave in a dark, cool place for about 4-6 weeks, stirring daily. After this time, strain the liquid and store in a dark bottle. Use according to the recommendations of a doctor or herbalist - usually a few drops a day, can be added to water or tea.

Juniper tincture is used in the treatment of urinary tract infections and digestive problems.

Juniper Oil

Ingredients:
- Fresh juniper berries
- Base oil (e.g., olive oil, coconut oil)

Preparation: Crush the juniper berries and put them in a jar, then pour over with the base oil so that all the berries are covered. Leave for 4-6 weeks in a dark, cool place. After this time, strain the oil and store in a dark bottle.

Juniper oil has antibacterial and antiviral properties and can be applied externally to treat minor skin infections.

Juniper Needle Syrup

Ingredients:
- 1 cup of fresh juniper needles
- 1 cup of sugar
- 2 cups of water

Preparation: In a large pot, add the juniper needles, sugar, and water. Bring to a boil, then reduce the heat and simmer for about an hour. Strain the syrup through a sieve into a clean jar.

Juniper needle syrup has antiseptic properties and can be used for gargling for throat pain and infections.

Juniper Needle Oil Macerate

Ingredients:
- 1 cup of fresh juniper needles
- 500 ml base oil (e.g., olive oil, coconut oil)

Preparation: Put the juniper needles in a jar, then pour over with the oil so that all needles are covered. Leave for 4-6 weeks in a dark, cool place. After this time, strain the oil and store in a dark bottle.

Juniper needle oil has antibacterial and antiviral properties, and can be applied externally to treat minor skin infections.

Juniper Bark Infusion

Ingredients:
- 1 teaspoon of finely chopped juniper bark
- 1 cup of hot water

Preparation: Pour the hot water over the juniper bark and leave it to infuse for about 15 minutes. Strain and drink once a day.

Juniper bark infusion helps to improve digestion and has a diuretic effect.

Cream from Juniper Berries

Ingredients:
- 1/2 cup juniper berries
- 1 cup coconut oil
- 1/4 cup beeswax
- 1/4 cup beeswax

Preparation: In a small pot, put juniper berries and coconut oil. Heat over low heat for about an hour, without allowing it to boil. After this time, strain the oil through a sieve into a clean jar, getting rid of the juniper berries. Add beeswax and avocado oil to the oil. Put the jar in a pot of water and heat on low heat until the wax dissolves, stirring all the time. When the wax has dissolved, remove the jar from the fire and let it cool. When the oil begins to thicken, you can mix it into a cream. Store in a cool place.

This cream has antibacterial and antiviral properties thanks to the juniper berries. It can be used for minor skin infections, as well as a body balm.

Phenolic Compounds: Juniper berries are rich in phenolic compounds, such as flavonoids and tannins, which have strong antioxidant properties.

Terpenes: Terpenes, such as pinene and camphene, have antibacterial, antiviral, and anti-inflammatory actions.

Vitamins: Juniper berries are a source of vitamins, especially vitamin C, which is a strong antioxidant.

Minerals: They also contain various minerals, such as calcium, magnesium, potassium, phosphorus, sodium, zinc, iron, and copper.

Fiber: They are a good source of fiber, which promotes digestive system health.

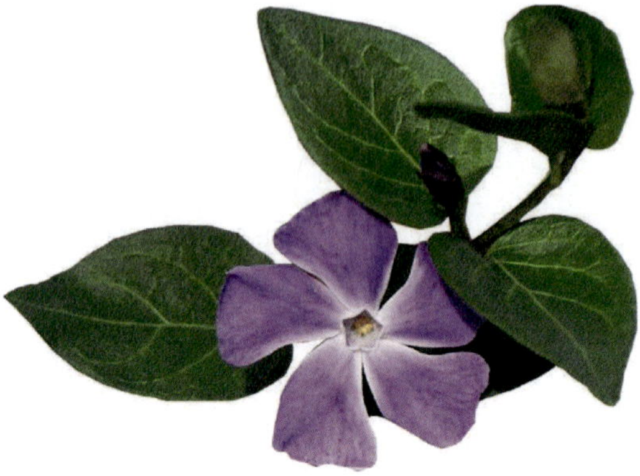

Lesser Periwinkle (Vinca minor)
This plant is appreciated in natural medicine for its alkaloid compounds, which help in the treatment of neurological problems and hypertension.

Although the use is wide, caution should be taken as the plant is toxic in large doses.

<u>Lesser Periwinkle Tea</u>

Ingredients:
- 1 teaspoon of dried lesser periwinkle leaves
- 1 cup of boiling water

Preparation: Pour boiling water over the dried periwinkle leaves. Allow to steep for about 10 minutes. Strain and consume 1-2 times a day.

This tea may help alleviate symptoms of hypertension and neurological problems.

Lesser Periwinkle Macerate for Skin Problems

Ingredients:
- A handful of fresh lesser periwinkle leaves
- 500 ml of olive oil (or other carrier oil, e.g., coconut oil)

Preparation: Wash the lesser periwinkle leaves and dry them. Transfer the leaves to a jar and pour oil over them. Store the jar in a warm, dark place for 4-6 weeks, regularly stirring the contents. After this time, strain the macerate through a sieve or gauze, store in a dark place.

Lesser periwinkle macerate can be used externally for skin problems such as hard-to-heal wounds, ulcers, burns, or skin inflammation.

Lesser Periwinkle Leaf Infusion for Rheumatic Pain Relief

Ingredients:
- 1 tablespoon of dried lesser periwinkle leaves
- 1 cup of boiling water

Preparation: Pour boiling water over the dried lesser periwinkle leaves. Cover and leave to infuse for about 10-15 minutes. Strain the infusion.

Use externally, soaking a bandage or gauze in the infusion and then applying to painful areas.

Alkaloids: This plant contains many different alkaloids, including vincamine, which is being studied for its potential brain health benefits.

Tannins: Lesser periwinkle is rich in tannins, which are known for their anti-inflammatory action and may help alleviate rheumatic pains.

Flavonoids: Flavonoids are potent antioxidants that can help protect the body from the harmful effects of free radicals.

Saponins: Saponins are another group of compounds that have various health actions, including potential anti-inflammatory effects.

Lesser Periwinkle (Vinca minor), also known as the small periwinkle, is a small, evergreen plant that was appreciated by the ancient inhabitants of Europe. It is rich in alkaloids such as vincamine and vinpocetine, which show promising effects in the treatment of various neurological conditions, including Alzheimer's disease, strokes, and memory problems. It is also used in the treatment of high blood pressure.

Periwinkle was appreciated for its medicinal properties by many ancient cultures, including the Vikings, who noticed its potential in combating inflammatory conditions and treating wounds.

However, this plant was used with due caution, given its toxicity.

In modern times, Lesser Periwinkle is still a valued element of phytotherapy. Scientific research confirms its benefits for brain and heart health.

At the same time, it is important to adhere to safe doses of this plant to avoid potential toxic effects.

Also today, periwinkle is often seen in gardens for its beautiful, blue flowers and evergreen leaves that add color even in the cooler months.

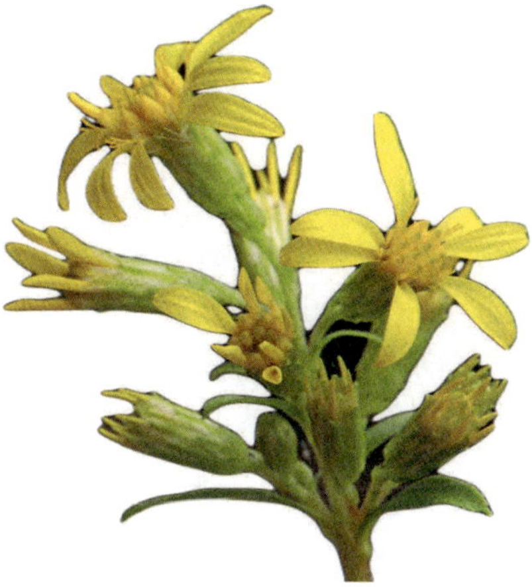

Common Goldenrod (Solidago virgaurea)
Known for its beneficial effect on the urinary system, especially in treating urinary tract infections.

Common Goldenrod Infusion

Ingredients:
- 2 tablespoons of dried common goldenrod
- 1 liter of boiling water

Preparation: Pour boiling water over the dried goldenrod and leave to infuse for about 10 minutes. Strain and drink 2-3 times a day.

Helpful in treating urinary tract infections, improving kidney function, and overall detoxification of the body.

Compresses with common goldenrod

Ingredients:
- A handful of fresh common goldenrod flowers
- Gauze or bandage

Preparation: Crush fresh goldenrod flowers and apply them to gauze or bandage. Apply to the painful area and secure.

Helpful in soothing skin inflammations, treating minor wounds, and burns.

Herbal blend with goldenrod

Ingredients:
- 1 tablespoon of dried goldenrod
- 1 tablespoon of dried chamomile flowers
- 1 tablespoon of dried peppermint leaves
- 1 liter of boiling water

Preparation: Pour boiling water over all the dried herbs and leave to infuse for about 15 minutes. Strain and drink 2-3 times a day.

This mixture can help soothe inflammation of the urinary tract, improve digestion, and provide relief in case of abdominal pain.

Goldenrod Ointment

Ingredients:
- 50 g fresh goldenrod flowers
- 200 ml of coconut oil
- 20 g of beeswax

Preparation: Place goldenrod flowers in a jar, add coconut oil and stir well. Put the jar in a pot with water and simmer on low heat for 2 hours (in a water bath). After 2 hours, strain the oil through a gauze into a clean jar, discarding the flower residues. Add beeswax to the oil and heat until the wax melts, stirring from time to time. Pour the hot mixture into jars and leave to cool.

Goldenrod ointment is a good skincare remedy, especially for eczema, psoriasis, irritations, or minor wounds. It can be applied to the skin 1-2 times a day.

Goldenrod Massage Oil

Ingredients:
- 1 cup of dried goldenrod flowers
- 1 cup of coconut oil or olive oil

Preparation: In a jar, place dried goldenrod flowers and cover them with the selected oil so that the flowers are completely covered. Close the jar and leave it in a warm, dark place for about 2 weeks, stirring the contents daily. After two weeks, strain the oil through a gauze into a clean jar, discarding the flower residues.

Goldenrod oil is excellent for massaging the skin, especially in places where there are muscle pains, spasms, or bruises. It can be used daily, massaging painful places.

Flavonoids: These are potent antioxidants that can help protect cells from damage by free radicals.

Triterpenes: These are chemical compounds that show a range of medicinal actions, including anti-inflammatory, antibacterial, and antiviral.

Phenolic acids: These compounds also act as antioxidants and may help protect the heart and blood vessels.

Polysaccharides: They can support the immune system and improve gut health.

Saponins: They have a diuretic effect, which may be particularly beneficial for people with urinary tract infections.

Mineral compounds: Goldenrod also contains small amounts of various minerals, such as potassium, calcium, magnesium, and phosphorus.

Vitamins: It also contains vitamin C, although its amount is not significant.

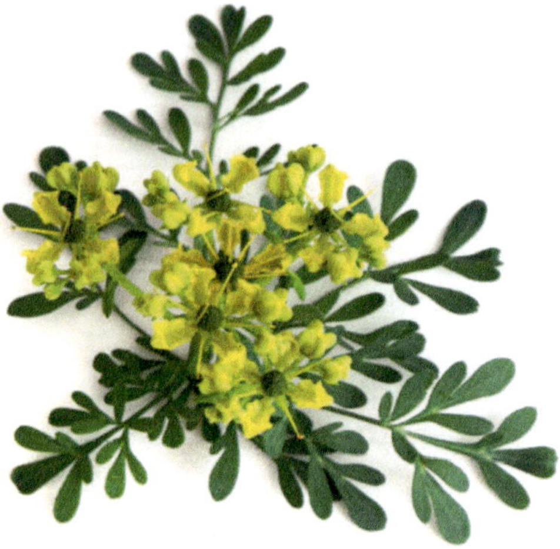

Common rue or Garden rue, (Ruta graveolens)
Ruta graveolens, also known as common rue or garden rue, is a plant that has been used in natural medicine for a long time. It was used to treat joint pains, insect bites, and eye problems, making rue an important part of rural medicine cabinets throughout Europe. It contains rutin - a compound from the flavonoid group, which has strong antioxidant and anti-inflammatory properties.

Rue is also used in aromatherapy due to its intense, specific scent. However, it should be noted that if used improperly, rue can be toxic.

<u>**Tincture of common rue for joint pain**</u>

Ingredients:
- 100g fresh rue leaves
- 500ml of 40-60% alcohol (e.g., spirit diluted to the appropriate concentration)

Preparation: Wash and dry the rue leaves thoroughly. Transfer the leaves to a jar and pour over the alcohol. Set aside for 2 weeks in a dark, cool place, stirring daily. After this time, strain the tincture and transfer to a dark bottle.

Apply externally, rubbing on the areas affected by pain.

Common rue compresses for insect bites

Ingredients:
- A few fresh rue leaves
- Bandage or gauze

Preparation: Wash the rue leaves thoroughly. Crush them to release the juice. Apply directly to the bite, securing with a bandage or gauze. Change the compresses every few hours.

Note: *Rue is phototoxic, which means it can cause skin irritation or burns when exposed to sunlight. Do not apply it to the skin before going out in the sun.*

Oil macerate of common rue

Ingredients:
- Fresh leaves of common ru
- Vegetable oil (for example, grapeseed oil, olive oil)

Preparation: Wash and dry the rue leaves. Put the leaves in a jar, not packing them too tightly. Pour the oil over the leaves so that they are completely covered. Close the jar and set aside for about 6 weeks in a warm, dark place. After this time, strain the oil through a thick cloth or coffee filter and transfer to a dark bottle.

Oil macerate of rue can be applied externally for aching joints, insect bites, or skin ailments.

Remember about the phototoxicity of rue - do not expose your skin to the sun after applying the macerate.

Alkaloids: Rue contains a range of different alkaloids, including rutin, which is thought to be responsible for many of its medicinal properties.

Coumarins: Rue is also rich in coumarins, which have strong antibacterial and antifungal properties.

Flavonoids: This plant also contains flavonoids, which are known antioxidants and may help protect the body from the harmful effects of free radicals.

Essential oils: Rue also contains many different essential oils, which may have antiseptic and anti-inflammatory effects.

Furanocoumarins: These compounds are present in many plants and have various medicinal properties, including antibacterial and anticancer activity.

Phenolic acids: These are natural compounds that have strong antioxidant properties and may help protect the body from oxidative damage.

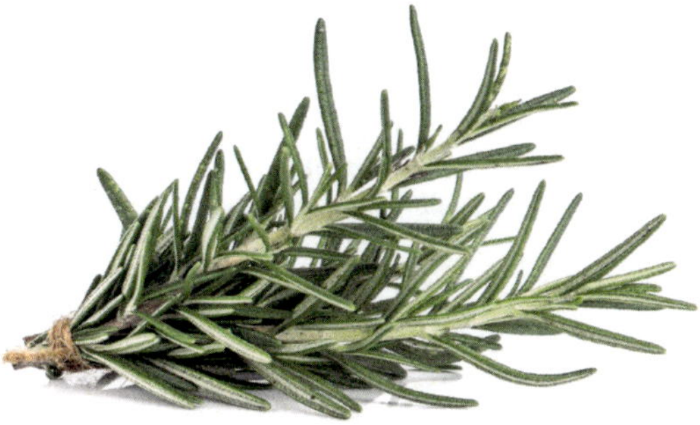

Rosemary (Rosmarinus officinalis)
Known for its antioxidant and anti-inflammatory properties. Often used in the treatment of digestive problems and to improve memory.

<u>Rosemary tea</u>

Ingredients:
- 1 teaspoon of dried rosemary leaves
- 1 cup of boiling water

Preparation: Pour the boiling water over the dried rosemary leaves and let them steep for about 10 minutes. Strain and drink 2-3 times a day.

Rosemary tea can help improve concentration, digestion, and can have a calming effect on stress.

Rosemary oil

Ingredients:
- Fresh rosemary leaves
- Oil (e.g., olive oil, coconut oil)
- Jar with a tight seal

Preparation: Place fresh rosemary leaves in the jar and cover with oil. Seal the jar tightly and set aside in a dark, cool place for 2-4 weeks. Strain through a sieve or gauze into a clean jar.

Rosemary oil can be applied topically to the skin, used for massage (helps with muscle pain), or added to a bath.

Rosemary hair rinse

Ingredients:
- 2 tablespoons of dried rosemary leaves
- 1 liter of water

Preparation: Pour a liter of water over two tablespoons of dried rosemary and simmer on low heat for 15-20 minutes. Remove from the heat and let cool, then strain.

Use the rosemary rinse after washing your hair, do not rinse it out. It will help to strengthen the hair and give it shine.

Rosemary face mask

Ingredients:
- 1 tablespoon of fresh rosemary leaves
- 1 teaspoon of honey
- 1 teaspoon of plain yogurt

Preparation: Chop the rosemary leaves. Mix with honey and yogurt. Apply the mask to cleansed face skin, avoiding the eye area. Leave on for 10-15 minutes. Rinse off with warm wat

Rosemary inhalation

Ingredients:
- A handful of fresh rosemary leaves
- A bowl of boiling water

Preparation: Add fresh rosemary leaves to a bowl of boiling water. Cover your head with a towel, creating a tent. Inhale the steam for about 10 minutes.

Rosemary facial tonic

Ingredients:
- A handful of fresh rosemary leaves
- 1 cup of water

Preparation: Pour boiling water over rosemary leaves. Brew for 15-20 minutes. After cooling down, strain the liquid. Store the toner in the refrigerator and use it to wash your face once a day.

Vitamins: Vitamin C: Rosemary is a good source of vitamin C, which is essential for the production of collagen, a protein that helps maintain the health of skin, tendons, blood vessels, and bones. Vitamin A: Also known as retinol, vitamin A is important for the health of vision, immune system, and reproduction. B Vitamins: Rosemary contains small amounts of B vitamins, such as folate, pyridoxine (B6), riboflavin, and thiamine (B1), which are necessary for proper metabolism in the body.

Minerals: Calcium: Calcium is necessary for healthy bones and teeth, as well as for the proper functioning of muscles and nerves.

Iron: Iron is necessary for the production of red blood cells and the transport of oxygen in the body.e.

Manganese: Manganese is important for bone health and helps in the metabolism of amino acids, cholesterol, glucose, and carbohydrates.

Magnesium: Magnesium is necessary for the proper functioning of the nervous system and muscles.

Antioxidants: Rosemary contains powerful antioxidants such as rosmarinic acid, carnosol, and eugenol, which help combat free radicals in the body.

Rosmarinic Acid: Rosmarinic acid has anti-inflammatory and anti-cancer properties. Essential Oils: Rosemary contains essential oils, which have many health benefits, including antibacterial and antifungal actions.

Rosemary is one of the most widely recognized herbs, long appreciated for both its culinary and medicinal properties. From ancient Celts and Vikings, through Druids, to contemporary botanists and pharmacists, rosemary is considered a health treasure trove.

Ancient Celts, known masters of herbs and natural healing, considered rosemary as one of the most important herbs. They used it for various purposes, from purifying rooms and using it as offerings for nature spirits, to utilizing it as an ingredient in healing elixirs. They believed that rosemary had the ability to protect against evil spirits, influencing their rituals and ceremonies.

The Vikings, known for utilizing herbs in their healing practices, also valued rosemary. They not only used it as a seasoning for food, but also as a remedy for various ailments, such as headaches, digestive problems, and even as a concentration-enhancing agent.

Today, in the world of pharmacy, rosemary is equally valued. Its main active ingredients, such as rosmarinol and rosmarinic acid, are researched for their potential health benefits, which include antioxidant, anti-inflammatory, anticancer, and neuroprotective actions. Furthermore, rosemary oil is often used in aromatherapy to alleviate stress and improve concentration.

While the methods of utilizing rosemary may vary depending on the culture and era, its universal health benefits make it an indispensable herb in both traditional and modern medicine.

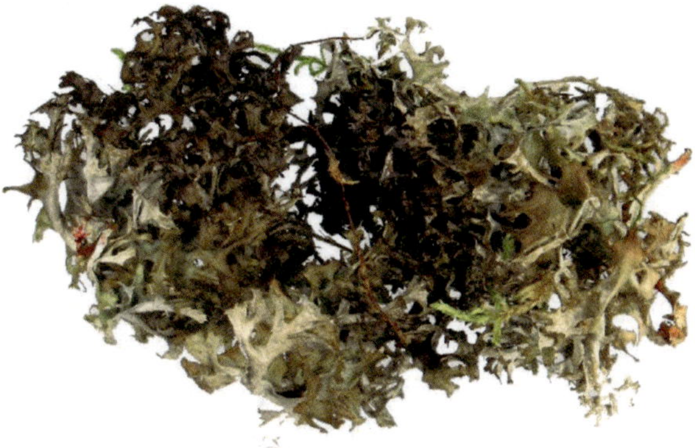

Icelandic Moss (Cetraria islandica)
This type of lichen is traditionally used in Iceland and other Nordic countries as an anti-inflammatory, antibacterial, and antiviral agent. It is also used to treat respiratory problems.

Icelandic Moss Infusion

Ingredients:
- 2 teaspoons of dried Icelandic moss
- 2 cups of water

Preparation: Pour water into a pot and bring it to a boil. Add the dried Icelandic moss to the boiling water. Reduce the heat to a minimum and let the herbs steep for about 15 minutes. After this time, strain the infusion and let it cool down. Drink 1-2 times a day, preferably after a meal.

This infusion helps in treating respiratory problems, such as a cough, sore throat, or asthma.

Icelandic Moss Honey

Ingredients:
- 1 cup of dried Icelandic moss
- 1 cup of honey

Preparation: Grind the dried Icelandic moss into a fine powder using a coffee grinder or blender. In a bowl, mix the moss powder with honey. Cover tightly and leave for 2 weeks in a dark, cool place, stirring daily. After two weeks, the honey is ready to eat. Store it in a tightly closed jar.

You can consume Icelandic moss honey by the spoonful once a day. The antibacterial and anti-inflammatory properties of this honey help in the treatment of respiratory tract infections and also improve overall health.

Icelandic Moss Tincture

Ingredients:
- 50 g of dried Icelandic moss
- 500 ml ml of spirit or vodka

Preparation: Place the dried Icelandic moss in a large glass jar. Add spirit or vodka. Close the jar and shake it to mix the ingredients. Leave it in a dark place for about 2 weeks, shaking the jar daily. After this time, strain the tincture through a coffee filter or gauze. Pour the tincture into bottles and store in a dark, cool place.

You can consume Icelandic moss tincture in small quantities (about 10 ml) once a day.

The anti-inflammatory and antibacterial properties of this tincture may help in the treatment of respiratory tract infections.

Icelandic Moss Syrup

Ingredients:
- 2 tablespoons of dried Icelandic moss
- 1 cup of water
- 1 cup of sugar

Preparation: Add water and sugar to a pot and then heat over medium heat until the sugar completely dissolves. Add the dried Icelandic moss to the pot and reduce the heat to a minimum. Simmer for about 30 minutes. After this time, strain the syrup through a coffee filter or gauze and let it cool down. Pour the syrup into a clean, glass bottle and store in the refrigerator.

Icelandic moss syrup can be added to tea, water, or other drinks to enhance their health properties. It acts anti-inflammatory and antibacterial, and also helps in treating respiratory system problems.

Icelandic Moss Compress

Ingredients:
- 2 tablespoons of dried Icelandic moss
- 1 cup of water

Preparation: Pour water into a pot and bring it to a boil. Add the dried Icelandic moss and reduce the heat. Simmer for about 15 minutes. After this time, strain the infusion and let it cool down. Soak a clean cloth or gauze in the infusion and apply to the affected areas of skin.

Compresses with an infusion of Icelandic moss are helpful in treating minor wounds, burns, skin inflammations, and bruises. They act antibacterial and anti-inflammatory.

Polysaccharides: Icelandic moss contains a rich amount of polysaccharides, including lichenin and isolichenin, which are known prebiotics and can contribute to gut health.

Usnic Acid: This is the primary bioactive component in Icelandic moss. Usnic acid is a strong antioxidant and has antibacterial, antiviral, and antifungal properties.

Fumarprotocetraric Acid: This compound has anti-inflammatory properties and is being studied for potential efficacy in treating certain diseases, such as arthritis.

Vitamin A: Icelandic moss contains Vitamin A, which is essential for eye health, skin health, and the immune system.

Vitamin B1 (Thiamine): Thiamine is essential for the proper functioning of the nervous system and glucose metabolism.

Minerals: Icelandic moss is a source of several minerals, such as manganese, magnesium, calcium, and zinc, which are necessary for the proper functioning of the body.

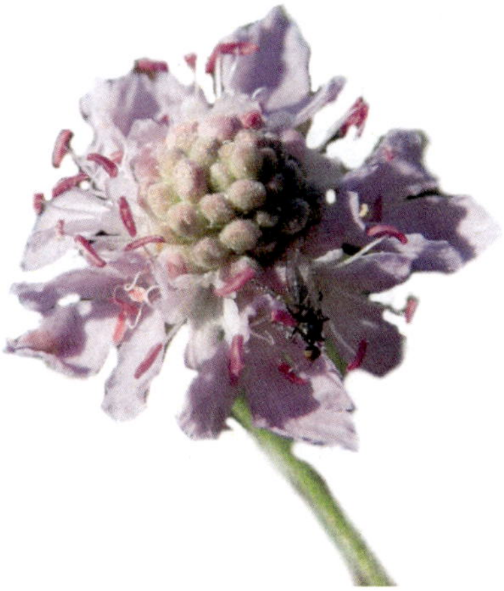

Sweet Scabious (Dianthus superbus)
This plant is used in Scandinavian folk medicine for the treatment of kidney diseases and urinary system issues.

Sweet Scabious Infusion

Ingredients:
- 2 teaspoons of dried sweet scabious flowers
- 2 cups of water

Preparation: Pour the water into a pot and bring to a boil. Add the dried sweet scabious flowers to the boiling water. Reduce the heat to low and let the herbs steep for about 10-15 minutes. Strain the infusion and let it cool. Drink 1-2 times a day, preferably after a meal.

The sweet scabious infusion is helpful in treating kidney diseases and urinary system issues. This herb acts as a diuretic, which helps cleanse the kidneys and the urinary system of toxins.

Sweet Scabious Tincture

Ingredients:
- 100 g of dried sweet scabious flowers
- 500 ml of vodka or spirit

Preparation: Place the dried sweet scabious flowers in a large, glass jar. Add vodka or spirit. Close the jar and leave it in a dark place for about 2 weeks, shaking the jar daily. After this time, strain the tincture and pour it into bottles. Store in a dark, cool place.

The sweet scabious tincture can be consumed in small amounts (about 10-15 ml) once a day. It helps support the health of the kidneys and urinary system, has diuretic and antibacterial effects.

Sweet Scabious Oil

Ingredients:
- 1 cup of dried sweet scabious flowers
- 2 cups of olive oil

Preparation: Place the dried sweet scabious flowers in a clean, dry jar. Pour in the olive oil, making sure the flowers are completely submerged. Close the jar and leave it in a warm place for about 4 weeks. Shake the jar every few days. After this time, strain the oil through a cheesecloth into a clean bottle. Store in a dark, cool place.

Sweet scabious oil can be applied externally to the skin to soothe inflammation and irritation. It also moisturizes and nourishes the skin.

Sweet Scabious Compress

Ingredients:
- A handful of dried sweet scabious flowers
- Warm water

Preparation: Place the dried flowers of sweet William in a bowl and add enough warm water to cover them. Let the flowers soak for about 10-15 minutes. After this time, drain the water and let the flowers cool to a temperature that is safe for the skin. Place the soaked flowers on a clean cloth or gauze and apply to the affected areas of the skin.

A compress made from sweet William can be applied externally to the affected areas of the skin to soothe irritation and inflammation.

Sweet William Syrup

Ingredients:
- 1 cup dried sweet William flowers
- 2 cups of water
- 1 cup of honey or sugar

Preparation: Pour water into a pot and add the dried sweet William flowers. Bring to a boil, then reduce the heat to a minimum and cook for about 15 minutes. Strain the infusion, return it to the pot, and add honey or sugar. Cook on low heat until the syrup thickens. Strain it again, then pour it into a sterile bottle and seal tightly. Store in the refrigerator.

Sweet William syrup is a good alternative to infusions and tinctures, especially for those who prefer a sweeter taste. The syrup can be added to tea or taken directly, a teaspoon twice a day.

Sweet William Hair Mask

Ingredients:
- 2 tablespoons of dried sweet william flowers
- 1 cup of water
- 1 tablespoon of coconut oil

Preparation: Pour water into a pot, add the dried sweet William flowers, and simmer for about 10 minutes. Strain the infusion and let it cool. Add the coconut oil to the infusion and mix well.

Apply the mask to your hair and scalp, leave it on for about 20 minutes, then wash your hair as usual. The soapwort hair mask helps nourish and moisturize the hair, as well as supports a healthy scalp. It can be used once a week.

Phenolic compounds: Soapwort is known for the presence of phenolic compounds, such as flavonoids, which act as strong antioxidants and can counteract damage caused by free radicals in the body.

Saponins: Soapwort contains saponins, which may have anti-inflammatory and antibacterial effects, as well as stimulate the urinary system, suggesting their diuretic properties.

In the medicinal tradition of ancient Scandinavian and European cultures, soapwort, called „the flower of the gods," adorned herbal pantries as a plant of inestimable values. Its power lay not only in the richness of its aroma, but also in its potent diuretic properties, which effectively supported the health of the kidneys and urinary system.

In the swirling centuries, this small but aromatic flower was also used in the production of luxury perfumes and high-quality cosmetics, emphasizing its universality and elegance.

Soapwort, though now often overlooked in favor of more well-known herbs, still has its worthy place in herbal medicine, constituting a bridge connecting us with the past. Discovering this plant is not only a return to the roots, but also a reminder of the richness of nature and the wisdom of our ancestors.

By getting to know such plants as soapwort, we have a chance to discover and appreciate the significance of traditional natural medicine and rediscover the value of often unjustly forgotten plants.

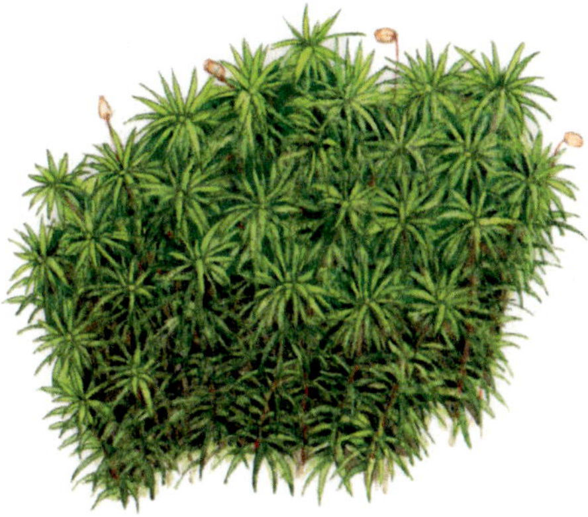

Polytrichum commune (Common Haircap Moss)
This is one of the most common species of moss in Europe and Scandinavia. Traditionally, it is used as an antiseptic and for wound healing. The moss hides incredible properties about which I will write to you, dear reader, below.

We are slowly approaching the end of our adventure but there are really still many revelations to come!

Moss collection: Choose healthy, green samples of Common Haircap Moss (Polytrichum commune). Avoid mosses that appear sick or discolored.

Only collect as much moss as you need, without completely destroying the local population.

Cleaning: Thoroughly clean the collected moss samples, remov

Drying: After cleaning, spread the moss on a flat surface that will allow it to dry. Leave it to dry completely, which can take from a few days to a week, depending on the conditions.

Storage: Store the dried moss in an airtight container until use.

Use as a dressing: Dressing preparation: Take an appropriate amount of dried moss and moisten it with clean water.

Application: Apply the moistened moss to the wound and gently wrap with a bandage to keep the moss in place.

Replacement: Change the dressing every few hours, or when it becomes dirty or dry.

Polysaccharides: Mosses, such as Common Haircap Moss, contain polysaccharides, which may have anti-inflammatory and anti-cancer effects.

Phytosterols: These are compounds naturally found in plants that can contribute to heart health.

Antioxidants: Mosses often contain compounds with antioxidant properties, which help fight free radicals in the body.

Antibacterial compounds: Some studies suggest that mosses may contain antibacterial compounds.

Antiviral compounds: Like antibacterial compounds, some studies suggest that mosses may contain antiviral compounds.

Minerals: Mosses, such as Common Haircap Moss, may contain trace amounts of minerals, such as potassium, magnesium, calcium, and others, which are essential for the proper functioning of the body.

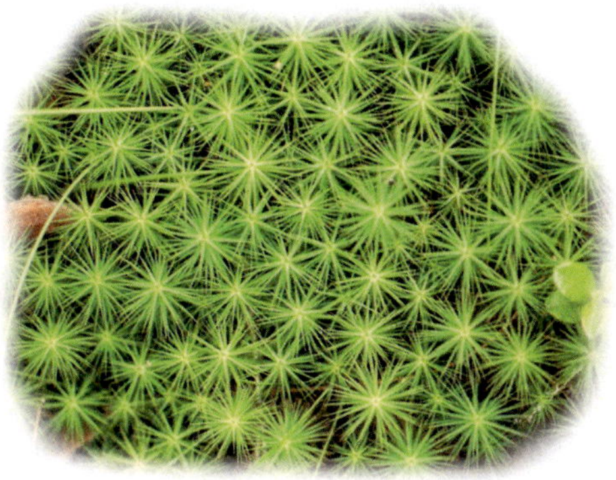

Polytrichum juniperinum (Juniper Haircap Moss)
Also known as juniper moss, this extraordinary plant has been an integral part of our natural pharmacy for centuries.

It is a species of moss that grows in diverse habitats worldwide, from desert fields to damp forests. It is known for its ability to survive in extreme conditions, which adds even more value in the context of traditional medicine.

Similar to Polytrichum commune, Juniper Haircap Moss (Polytrichum juniperinum) is used in traditional folk medicine, mainly as an antiseptic and for wound healing.

Preparing moss for dressings

Moss collection: Collect healthy, green samples of Juniper Haircap Moss.

Avoid mosses that appear sick or discolored.

Collect only as much moss as you need, without destroying the entire local population.

Cleaning: Thoroughly clean the collected moss samples, removing any visible impurities.

Drying: After cleaning, spread the moss on a flat surface that will allow it to dry. Leave it to dry completely, which can take from a few days to a week, depending on the conditions.

Storage: Store the dried moss in an airtight container until use.

Use as a dressing:
Dressing preparation: Take an appropriate amount of dried moss and moisten it with clean water.

Application: Apply the moistened moss to the wound and gently wrap with a bandage to keep the moss in place.

Replacement: Change the dressing every few hours, or when it becomes dirty or dry.

Polysaccharides: Juniper Haircap Moss, like many other moss species, contains polysaccharides, which may have anti-inflammatory and anti-cancer effects.

Phytosterols: These are compounds naturally found in plants, including Juniper Haircap Moss. They may contribute to improved heart health by lowering levels of bad LDL cholesterol.

Antioxidants: Mosses, like Juniper Haircap Moss, often contain compounds with antioxidant properties, which help combat harmful free radicals in the body.

Antibacterial compounds: Although this requires further research, some indicate that Juniper Haircap Moss may contain compounds with potential antibacterial activity.

Antiviral compounds: Similar to antibacterial compounds, research suggests that mosses may contain antiviral compounds, although specifically for Juniper Haircap Moss, this requires further research.

Minerals: Juniper Haircap Moss may contain trace amounts of minerals such as potassium, magnesium, calcium, and others, which are crucial for the proper functioning of the body.

In natural medicine, Juniper Haircap Moss was often used as an effective antibacterial agent.

Its unique medicinal properties were appreciated by ancient communities who used it to accelerate wound healing, reduce inflammation, and as a support in the fight against bacterial infections.

Thanks to its versatility and availability, this plant gained recognition in various cultures, from ancient druids to Nordic tribes.

Although its significance in today's medicine is a lesser-known fact, it still constitutes an essential component of some herbal preparations, and research on its properties continues, discovering more and more potential uses of Juniper Haircap Moss in the context of health and wellness.

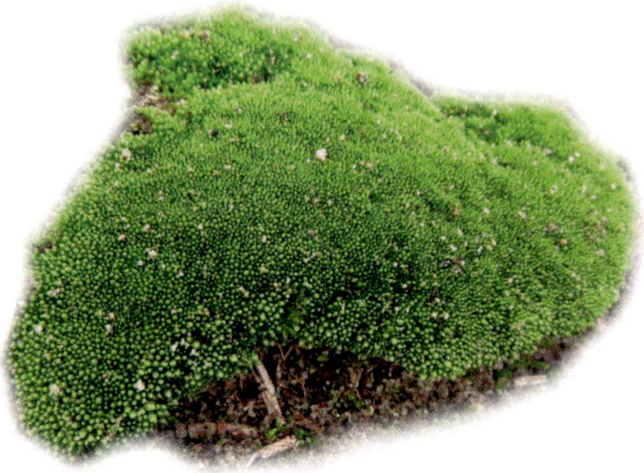

Bryum argenteum (Silver Moss)
This species of moss is used in folk medicine to treat burns and other skin ailments.

Infusion for burns and skin conditions

Ingredients:
- 2 tablespoons of Silver Moss (Bryum argenteum)
- 1 cup of boiling water

Preparation: Collect 2 tablespoons of Silver Moss. Make sure it's clean and not contaminated. Pour boiling water into a vessel, then add the moss to it. Leave the infusion to brew for about 15 minutes. Strain the infusion, removing any remnants of the moss. Soak a clean cloth or sponge in the infusion and apply it to burns or skin areas with ailments.

<u>Ointment for burns and skin conditions</u>

Ingredients:
- 2 tablespoons of Silver Moss (Bryum argenteum)
- 1 cup of coconut oil or olive oil
- 1/4 cup of beeswax

Preparation: Collect 2 tablespoons of Silver Moss. Make sure it's clean and not contaminated. Pour oil into a pot and heat on low heat. Add moss to the oil and simmer on low heat for about 1 hour. Strain the oil through a sieve into another container, removing the remnants of the moss. Pour beeswax into the oil and heat until the wax melts. After the wax has melted, pour the ointment into a clean jar and leave it to cool down.

<u>Silver Moss (Bryum argenteum) Tincture for skin problems</u>

Ingredients:
- 1 cup of Silver Moss (Bryum argenteum)
- 2 cups of 70% alcohol

Preparation: Collect clean, uncontaminated Silver Moss. Place the moss in a clean jar. Pour alcohol over it so that the moss is completely covered. Close the jar and store it in a dark, cool place for 4-6 weeks, stirring the contents every few days. After this time, strain the tincture through a sieve, separating the remnants of the moss.

The tincture can be used externally, by soaking a clean cloth or sponge and applying it to burns, skin inflammations, or areas with bacterial infections.

Silver Moss (Bryum argenteum) Mouth Rinse Mixture

Ingredients:
- 2 tablespoons of Silver Moss (Bryum argenteum)
- 1 cup of water

Preparation: Collect 2 tablespoons of Silver Moss, ensuring it is clean and uncontaminated. Pour water into a container, then add the moss to it. Leave it to steep for about 15 minutes. Strain the mixture, removing remnants of the moss.

The mixture can be used for mouth rinsing to alleviate symptoms of gum inflammation, bacterial infections, or throat inflammation.

Polysaccharides: Like other mosses, Bryum argenteum contains polysaccharides, which are being studied for potential anti-inflammatory and immunomodulatory properties.

Antioxidants: Mosses often contain compounds with antioxidant properties, which can help protect the body from the harmful effects of free radicals.

Antibacterial and antiviral compounds: Some research suggests that mosses, including Bryum argenteum, may contain compounds with potential antibacterial and antiviral activity.

Minerals: Mosses, depending on where they grow, can accumulate various minerals from their environment.

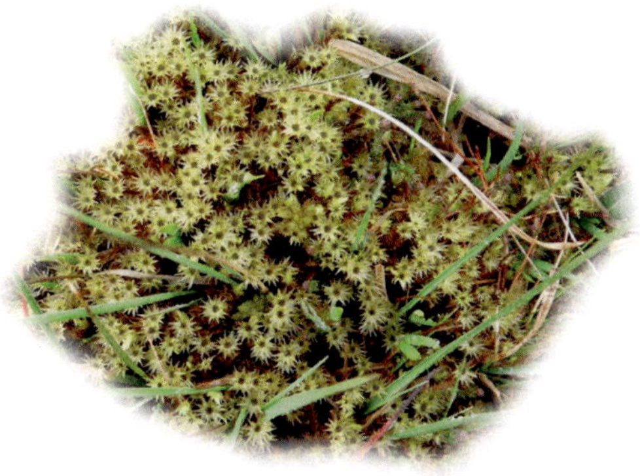

Aulacomnium palustre (Bog haircap moss)
Used for centuries as a potent anti-inflammatory and antibacterial agent, this remarkable species of moss played a pivotal role in the traditional medicine of ancient European civilizations. It is commonly found in regions with a humid climate, such as Ireland or Norway, and its therapeutic properties were well-known to both the ancient Celts and the Vikings.

The ancient communities, harnessing the benefits of nature, frequently employed bog haircap moss to treat a wide array of ailments. Its innate anti-inflammatory and antibacterial properties proved effective in combatting infections and inflammations.
Moreover, it was applied externally to address wounds, bites, and skin inflammations, serving as a natural, accessible, and efficacious medicinal remedy.

Antibacterial action: Similar to many other moss species, Aulacomnium palustre demonstrates potential antibacterial activity. Although detailed studies on its effectiveness against specific pathogens are limited, the general antibacterial action of mosses may indicate potential use against a wide spectrum of bacteria.

Anti-inflammatory action: Mosses, including Aulacomnium palustre, contain polysaccharides and other compounds that may have anti-inflammatory effects. This can be particularly beneficial in treating inflammatory skin conditions such as eczema, acne, or burns, but also in treating other inflammatory conditions in the body.

Infusion with Aulacomnium palustre for inflammatory skin conditions

Ingredients:
- 2 tablespoons of dried Aulacomnium palustre moss
- 500 ml of water

Preparation: Pour the water into a small pot and bring it to a boil. Once the water starts boiling, add the dried moss and reduce the heat. Simmer on low heat for 10 minutes. After this time, strain the infusion into a glass through a sieve or coffee filter and let it cool. After cooling, the infusion can be used as a rinse for skin with inflammatory problems. Apply the rinse to the skin using a cotton pad 2-3 times a day.

Ointment with Aulacomnium palustre for inflammatory skin conditions

Ingredients:
- 4 tablespoons of dried Aulacomnium palustre moss
- 200 g of shea butter

Preparation: Place the shea butter in a bowl and melt it in a water bath. When the shea butter is completely melted, add the dried moss and stir to combine. Allow the mixture to cool, and then place it in the refrigerator to solidify. Store the ointment in a tightly sealed container in a cool place.

The Aulacomnium palustre ointment can be applied 2-3 times a day to skin with inflammatory problems.

Aulacomnium palustre Infusion for Drinking

Ingredients:
- 1 teaspoon of dried Aulacomnium palustre moss
- 1 cup of hot water

Preparation: Pour the hot water into a cup with the dried moss. Let the infusion steep for 10 minutes. After this time, strain the infusion through a sieve into another cup. The Aulacomnium palustre infusion can be drunk up to 3 times a day.

This helps alleviate inflammatory conditions of the mucous membranes of the digestive system.

Aulacomnium palustre Elixir for Immunity Boost

Ingredients:
- 2 tablespoons of dried Aulacomnium palustre moss
- 500 ml of honey

Preparation: In a small pot, heat the honey on low heat, but do not let it boil. Add the dried moss to the honey and stir. Leave on low heat for 30 minutes, stirring regularly. After this time, strain the honey through a sieve or coffee filter into a clean jar.

The Aulacomnium palustre elixir can be consumed daily, by tablespoon, to support the immune system.iczny.

Aulacomnium palustre Paste for Skin Conditions

Ingredients:
- 1 tablespoon of dried Aulacomnium palustre moss
- 1 tablespoon of glycerin

Preparation: In a small bowl, mix the dried Aulacomnium palustre moss with glycerin to form a consistent paste. Apply the paste to areas with skin conditions. Leave it on the skin for 15-20 minutes, and then rinse off with lukewarm water.

Aulacomnium palustre Oil for Massage

Ingredients:
- 2 tablespoons of dried Aulacomnium palustre moss
- 500 ml of coconut oil

Preparation: In a small pot, heat the coconut oil on low heat. Add the dried moss to the oil and stir. Cook on low heat for 30 minutes. After this time, strain the oil through a sieve or coffee filter into a clean bottle.

The Aulacomnium palustre oil can be used as a massage oil for aching muscles.

Polysaccharides: Mosses, such as Aulacomnium palustre, contain polysaccharides that may have anti-inflammatory properties.

Phytosterols: These are compounds naturally occurring in plants that may contribute to heart health.

Antioxidants: Mosses often contain compounds with antioxidant properties that help fight free radicals in the body.

Antibacterial compounds: Some research suggests that mosses may contain compounds with antibacterial properties.

Minerals: Mosses, such as Aulacomnium palustre, may contain trace amounts of minerals such as potassium, magnesium, calcium, and others.

Antiviral compounds: Similarly to antibacterial compounds, some research suggests that mosses may contain antiviral compounds.

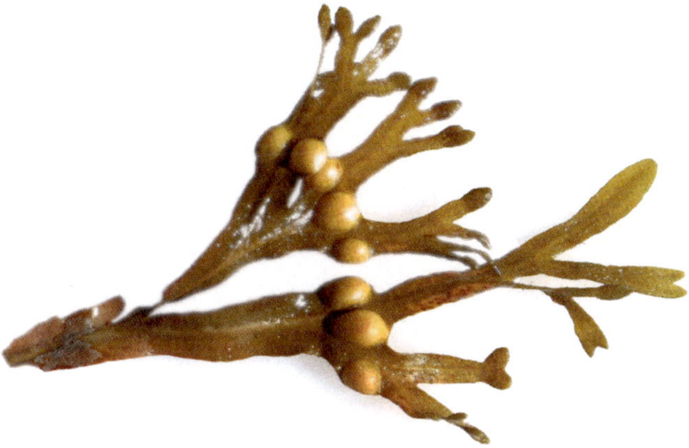

Bladderwrack (Fucus vesiculosus)
This is one of the most frequently used seaweeds in traditional medicine. It contains iodine, which is necessary for the proper functioning of the thyroid. Traditionally, it is used to treat thyroid problems and obesity.

<u>Decoction of Bladderwrack for Improving Thyroid Function</u>

Ingredients:
- 2 tablespoons of dried bladderwrack
- 2 cups of water

Preparation: Add water and bladderwrack to the pot. Simmer on low heat for about 20 minutes. After this time, strain the infusion and let it cool down. Drink two cups a day, preferably before meals.

A decoction of bladderwrack is traditionally used to treat thyroid problems associated with iodine deficiency.

Bladderwrack Drink for Weight Loss

Ingredients:

- 1 tablespoon of dried bladderwrack
- cup of warm water
- teaspoon of honey (optional)

Preparation: Pour warm water over the bladderwrack and leave it for 10 minutes. After this time, strain the drink and add a teaspoon of honey to improve the taste, if you want. Drink twice a day, preferably before meals.

A bladderwrack drink is traditionally used to support weight loss. The polysaccharides contained in it can help create a sense of fullness.

Bladderwrack Mask for Acne

Ingredients:

- 1 tablespoon of dried bladderwrack
- 1 teaspoon of honey
- Water

Preparation: Grind the dried bladderwrack to a powder in a coffee grinder or blender. In a bowl, mix the powder with honey, adding eno-ugh water to make a paste. Apply to the face, avoiding the eye area, and leave on for 15-20 minutes. After this time, rinse the mask off with warm water.

Bladderwrack has antiseptic properties that can help fight acne. Honey additionally moisturizes the skin and has anti-inflammatory effects.

Bladderwrack Bath for Joint Pain

Ingredients:

- 2 cups of dried bladderwrack
- A comfortable bathtub

Preparation: Put the dried bladderwrack in a bag made of water-permeable material (e.g., cotton). Fill the bathtub with warm water and place the bag with bladderwrack in the tub. Leave it for 20-30 minutes so that the active substances from the bladderwrack pass into the water. Immerse yourself in the bath for 15-20 minutes.

A bath with bladderwrack can help relieve joint and muscle pain. It has relaxing and anti-inflammatory effects.

Bladderwrack Elixir for Immunity Boosting

Ingredients:
- 1 cup of dried bladderwrack
- 1 liter of water
- 1 lemon
- Honey to taste

Preparation: Add water and dried bladderwrack to a large pot. Bring to a boil, then reduce the heat and simmer for 20-30 minutes. After this time, strain the drink through a sieve, removing the bladderwrack. Pour the liquid back into the pot. Add the juice of a lemon and honey to taste. Heat on medium heat, stirring until the honey dissolves. Allow the elixir to cool, then store it in the refrigerator.
The bladderwrack elixir can be drunk daily to increase immunity. Bladderwrack contains a large amount of iodine, which is necessary for the proper functioning of the thyroid, as well as antioxidants, which can help fight free radicals. Lemon adds vitamin C, and honey has antibacterial action.arczycy, a także przeciwutleniacze, które mogą pomóc w walce z wolnymi rodnikami. Cytryna dodaje witaminy C, a miód ma działanie antybakteryjne.

Bladderwrack, Mint, and Lemon Balm Elixir

Ingredients:
- 2 tablespoons of dried bladderwrack
- 1 liter of water
- 1 cup of fresh mint leaves
- 1 cup of fresh lemon balm leaves
- 2 tablespoons of honey (optional)

Preparation: Add the dried bladderwrack, mint, and lemon balm to a pot of water. Turn on the heat and bring to a boil. Once the water begins to boil, reduce the heat to a minimum and simmer for about 20 minutes. After this time, strain the mixture, discarding the bladderwrack, mint, and lemon balm. When the liquid has cooled, add honey to taste if desired. Stir well until the honey is completely dissolved.

This elixir combines the calming properties of mint and lemon balm with the nutrient-richness of bladderwrack, creating a natural remedy to help cope with stress. Drink a cup of this elixir in the evening to relax after a long day.

Lodine is essential for thyroid health, and bladderwrack is one of the best natural sources of this mineral. Iodine is key to the production of thyroid hormones, which regulate many important bodily functions, including metabolic rate.

Polysaccharides: Bladderwrack contains polysaccharides such as fucoidan and alginates, which have many potential health benefits, including anti-inflammatory, anti-cancer, and anti-diabetic effects.

Polyphenols: These compounds have strong antioxidant properties, which can help fight free radicals and protect the body from the harmful effects of oxidative stress.

Vitamins and Minerals: Bladderwrack also contains a range of other vitamins and minerals, including vitamins A, C, E, and B, as well as minerals such as calcium, magnesium, zinc, selenium, and copper.

Alginic Acid: Alginic acid, which is present in bladderwrack, is known for its ability to bind heavy metals and remove them from the body. It can also help regulate blood cholesterol levels.

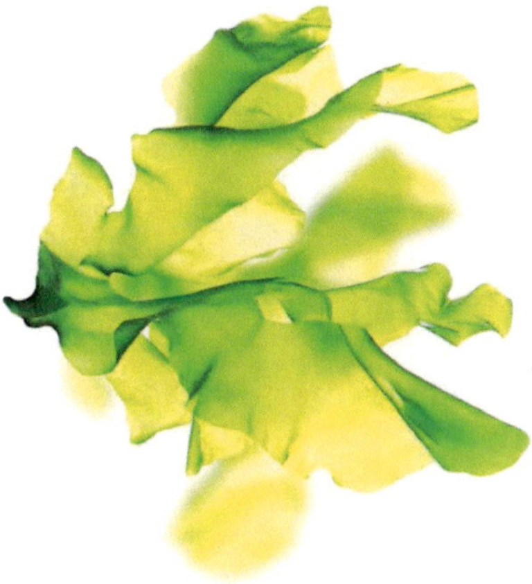

Sea Lettuce (Ulva lactuca)
This is a green algae known for its high content of protein, iron, and B vitamins.

Sea Lettuce Infusion

Ingredients:
- 1 tablespoon dried sea lettuce (Ulva lactuca)
- 1 cup of hot water

Preparation: Pour hot water over the dried sea lettuce. Leave the infusion for 10-15 minutes, then strain. The sea lettuce infusion can be drunk 1-2 times a day. It is nutritious and strengthening for the body.

Sea Lettuce Ointment

Ingredients:
- 1 cup of fresh sea lettuce (Ulva lactuca)
- 1 cup of coconut oil
- 1/4 cup of beeswax

Preparation: Wash the sea lettuce thoroughly, dry it, and chop it finely. In a pot over low heat, heat the coconut oil, add the sea lettuce. Stir until the sea lettuce has completely dissolved. Add the beeswax and stir until the wax has melted. Remove the pot from the heat and strain the mixture into a clean jar. Allow the ointment to cool.

The sea lettuce ointment can be applied externally to the skin for moisturizing and regeneration. Due to its high content of protein, iron, and B vitamins, the ointment may help treat minor irritations and improve the overall condition of the skin.

Protein: Sea lettuce is known for its high protein content, which is necessary for the construction and regeneration of cells in the body.

Vitamins: Sea lettuce contains large amounts of vitamins, especially B-group vitamins. These vitamins are necessary for the proper functioning of the nervous system and metabolism.

Minerals: Sea lettuce is rich in various minerals, such as iron, potassium, magnesium, and calcium. These minerals are necessary for the proper functioning of the body, including for healthy bones and teeth, proper blood clotting, and maintaining normal blood pressure.

Fiber: Sea lettuce is also a source of fiber, which helps maintain the health of the digestive system and can contribute to maintaining a healthy weight.

Bioactive compounds: Sea lettuce also contains various bioactive compounds, such as polyphenols and carotenoids, which are strong antioxidants and can help protect the body from damage caused by free radicals.

Omega-3 Fatty Acid: Sea lettuce also contains Omega-3 fatty acid, which is necessary for heart and brain health.

Sea lettuce is a species of green algae that has long been valued in natural medicine for its unique health benefits.

Rich in proteins, iron, B vitamins, and fiber, it was often used as food, but also as a medicinal remedy in the treatment of various ailments. In Viking times, it was a key component of the diet, providing valuable nutrients and supporting health.

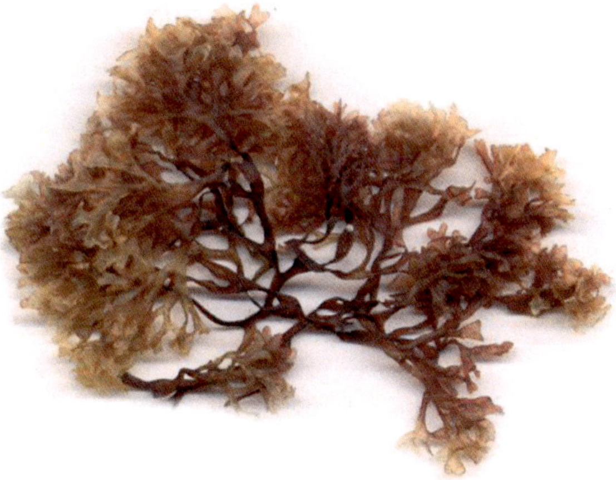

Irish Moss Alg (Chondrus crispus)
It is used in the food industry as a gelling agent. It contains numerous minerals and is rich in protein.

Irish Moss Alg Infusion

Ingredients:
- 2 tablespoons of dried Irish moss
- 1 liter of water

Preparation: Pour boiling water over the dried Irish moss and let it steep for about 20 minutes. After this time, strain the infusion and drink it. This infusion is known for its antibacterial and antiviral properties.

Irish Moss Alg Compress

Ingredients:
- 2 tablespoons of dried Irish moss
- 1 liter of water

Preparation: Pour boiling water over the dried Irish moss and let it steep for about 20 minutes. After this time, strain the liquid, soak a clean cloth in it, and apply to the area that needs treatment.

This compress is known for its anti-inflammatory action and can be used to treat various skin conditions.

Irish Moss Jelly

Ingredients:
- 1 cup of dried Irish moss
- 3 cups of water
- Honey to taste

Preparation: Pour water over the dried Irish moss and simmer for about 30 minutes. After this time, strain the liquid and add honey to taste. Leave the jelly to cool down, then store it in the fridge.

Irish moss jelly is rich in minerals and vitamins, making it a healthy dessert.

Irish Moss Ointment

Ingredients:
- 1 cup of dried Irish moss
- 2 cups of coconut oil
- 1/4 cup of beeswax

Preparation: First, make a decoction of Irish moss. Pour 2 cups of boiling water over the dried Irish moss and let it steep for about 20 minutes

After this time, strain the decoction and grind the Irish moss into a fine powder. Heat the coconut oil in a saucepan. Add the ground Irish moss to it and mix well. Add beeswax and keep stirring until the wax is completely melted. Remove the saucepan from the heat and let the ointment cool. Pour it into a clean jar and store in a cool place.

Such ointment has moisturizing and soothing effects.

It acts anti-inflammatory and antibacterial.

It's perfect for skin care, especially in case of problems like eczema or psoriasis.

Vitamin A: this is an important antioxidant that helps maintain the health of skin and eyes.

B Vitamins: these vitamins help the body convert food into energy and support the health of the nervous system.

Vitamin C: has strong antioxidant properties, supports the immune system and is important for collagen production.

Vitamin K: this vitamin is essential for proper blood clotting.

Iodine: is essential for the proper functioning of the thyroid.

Potassium: this mineral is important for proper muscle function and maintaining fluid balance in the body.

Calcium: is a key component for bone and teeth health. Magnesium: this mineral is important for many functions in the body, including proper muscle function and the nervous system.

Iron: is crucial for the production of hemoglobin, a protein that carries oxygen in red blood cells.

Proteins: Chondrus crispus contains several amino acids, which are the building blocks of proteins. Proteins are essential for building and repairing tissues in the body.

Fiber: aids in digestion and can contribute to maintaining a healthy weight.

Antioxidants: Contains numerous compounds with antioxidant activity that neutralize harmful free radicals in the body.

Polysaccharides: These include carrageenans, which have anti-inflammatory and immunomodulatory effects.

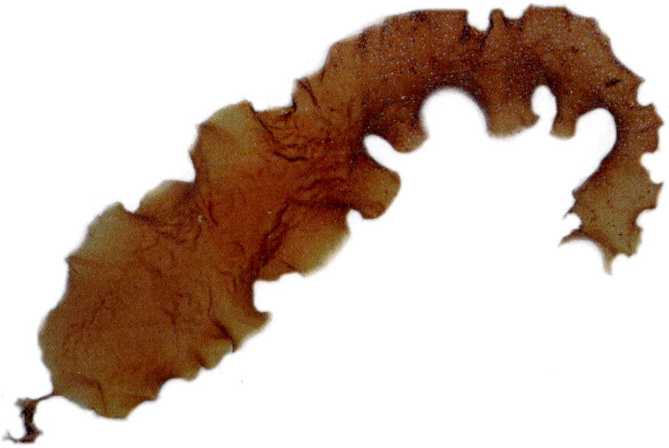

Saccharina latissima (Laminaria saccharina))
These algae are rich in iodine, which is necessary for the proper functioning of the thyroid. They are also a source of other minerals such as potassium, iron, calcium, and zinc.

Sargassum Muticum Infusion

Ingredients:
- 2 tablespoons of dried Sargassum muticum
- 1 liter of water

Preparation: Start by thoroughly washing the dried Sargassum muticum under running water to remove any impurities. Place 2 tablespoons of seaweed in a thermos. Pour boiling water over the algae and tightly close the thermos. Allow the seaweed to steep for about 20 minutes. After this time, the infusion is ready to consume.

You can drink it directly or strain it if you prefer an infusion without plant parts. It is recommended to consume the infusion fresh, ideally within 1-2 hours of preparation.

Immune Boost: Regular consumption of Sargassum muticum infusion can help in building a strong immune defense, effectively supporting the body in fighting pathogens.

Improvement of Skin Condition: External application of this infusion, for example in the form of baths or compresses, has the potential to improve various skin ailments such as skin inflammation, eczema, acne, or psoriasis.

Digestive Disorders: In traditional Asian medicine, Sargassum muticum infusion is used to alleviate digestive ailments such as irregular bowel movements or diarrhea..

Neutralization of Free Radicals: Seaweeds are known for their rich content of antioxidants that can counteract cellular damage caused by free radicals, thereby reducing oxidative stress.

Sargassum Muticum Ointmen

Ingredients:

- 1 cup of dried Sargassum muticum
- 2 cups of coconut oil (you can also use olive oil)
- 1/4 cup of beeswax

Preparation: First, prepare the Sargassum muticum. Wash the dried seaweed under running water to remove any impurities. Then grind the seaweed into a fine powder using a coffee grinder or blender. The ground seaweed should have a consistency similar to flour. Proceed to prepare the oil. In a large pot on medium heat, warm the coconut oil. When the oil has melted and is warm, add the ground seaweed to it. Stir to combine the oil with the seaweed well. Cook the oil and seaweed mixture on low heat for about 2-3 hours, stirring regularly. After this time, add the beeswax to the pot. Stir until the wax is completely dissolved. When the wax is completely dissolved, strain the mixture through a fine sieve or cloth into a clean jar, removing any seaweed residues.

Allow the ointment to cool. When the ointment begins to solidify, close the jar and store it in a cool place.

Sargassum Muticum ointment can be applied topically to the skin to alleviate various skin problems. It can help treat skin dryness, rashes, eczema, psoriasis, and even burns

Additionally, this ointment can help reduce inflammation and pain associated with various skin ailments. Use the ointment 1-2 times a day, gently rubbing it into the skin.

Sargassum Muticum Tincture

Ingredients:
- 1 cup of dried Sargassum muticum
- 1 liter of alcohol (vodka, rum, or gin)

Preparation: Rinse the dried Sargassum muticum in cold water, then dry. Place the dried Sargassum muticum into a large jar with a thick, airtight lid. Add the alcohol to the jar, making sure that all the Sargassum is submerged. Screw on the jar and keep it in a dark, cool place for at least two weeks, shaking the contents daily. After two weeks, strain the liquid through a fine sieve or coffee filter into a clean container. The tincture should be clear and transparent.

The tincture is rich in antioxidants and can be consumed orally for overall health improvement. It is recommended to drink 1-2 teaspoons daily.

Sargassum Muticum Poultice

Ingredients:
- 1 cup of dried Sargassum muticum
- Water

Preparation: Rinse the dried Sargassum muticum in cold water. Place the Sargassum in a bowl and cover it with warm water. Allow it to soak for at least 30 minutes until it becomes soft. After soaking, strain the Sargassum and place it on a clean cotton cloth.

Fold the cloth with Sargassum onto the area that requires treatment. This poultice is known for its anti-inflammatory properties and can be used to treat various skin conditions such as eczema or psoriasis.

Protein: Sargassum muticum is rich in proteins, which are necessary for the construction and regeneration of cells in the body.

Vitamins: Sargassum muticum contains high amounts of vitamins, especially those of the B group, which are necessary for the proper functioning of the nervous system and metabolism.

Minerals: Sargassum muticum is rich in various minerals, such as iodine, potassium, magnesium, and calcium. These minerals are essential for the proper functioning of the body, including for healthy bones and teeth, proper blood clotting, and maintaining proper blood pressure.

Polysaccharides: Sargassum muticum contains high amounts of polysaccharides, including fucoidan and alginate. These substances have potential anti-cancer and antiviral actions.

Antioxidants: Sargassum muticum is rich in natural antioxidants, which help protect the body's cells from damage caused by free radicals.

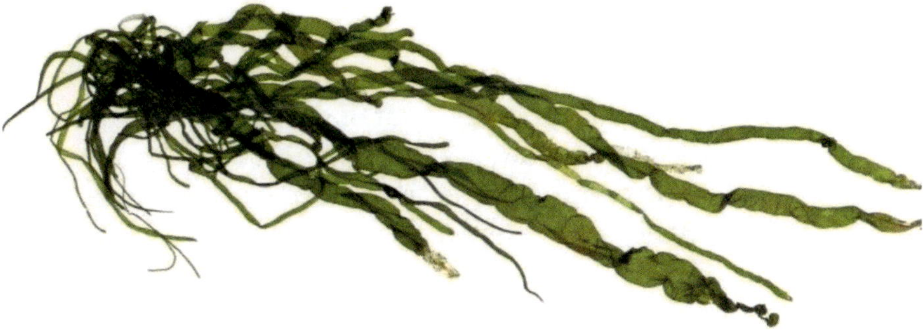

Enteromorpha intestinalis
This species is rich in protein, fiber, vitamins, and minerals. Traditionally, it is used as a detoxifying and anti-inflammatory agent..

Infusion of Enteromorpha intestinalis

Ingredients:
- 2 tablespoons of dried Enteromorpha intestinalis
- 1 liter of water

Preparation: Pour boiling water over the dried Enteromorpha intestinalis. Leave the infusion for about 20 minutes to fully extract the nutritional and medicinal ingredients. After this time, strain the infusion through a sieve into another container, getting rid of the seaweed residue. The infusion is ready to drink. You can drink it 2-3 times a day.

The Enteromorpha intestinalis infusion is rich in protein, fiber, vitamins, and minerals. It is used as a detoxifying agent, aids digestion, and has anti-inflammatory properties.

Enteromorpha intestinalis Poultice

Ingredients:
- 2 tablespoons of dried Enteromorpha intestinalis
- 1 liter of water

Preparation: Pour boiling water over the dried Enteromorpha intestinalis. Leave the infusion for about 20 minutes to fully extract the nutritional and medicinal ingredients. After this time, strain the infusion through a sieve into another container, getting rid of the seaweed residue. Soak a clean cloth in the infusion and apply to the skin as a poultice. The Enteromorpha intestinalis poultice has anti-inflammatory and detoxifying properties.

It can be used to treat various skin conditions, such as eczema, acne, as well as irritations and burns.

Enteromorpha intestinalis Elixir

Ingredients:
- 50 g dried enteromorpha intestinalis
- 500 ml alcohol (40-60%, for example vodka)

Preparation: Place the dried Enteromorpha intestinalis in a jar. Cover with alcohol so that the entire seaweed is covered. Close the jar and leave in a dark place for 2-3 weeks, stirring the contents daily. After this time, strain the elixir through a sieve or densely woven cloth, store in a dark bottle.

The Enteromorpha intestinalis elixir has detoxifying and anti-inflammatory properties. It can be used internally (1-2 teaspoons a day) to support digestion and cleanse the body, or externally on the skin to alleviate inflammation and irritation.

Enteromorpha Intestinalis Oil

Ingredients:
- 50 g dried enteromorpha intestinalis
- 500 ml ml oil (e.g., olive oil, coconut oil)

Preparation: Place the dried Enteromorpha intestinalis in a jar. Pour in the oil so that the entirety is well covered. Close the jar and leave it in a dark, cool place for 4-6 weeks. After this time, strain the oil through a sieve or densely woven cloth, and store it in a dark bottle.

The Enteromorpha intestinalis oil moisturizes and regenerates the skin. It can be used on all kinds of irritations and skin inflammations. You can use it like a normal body oil, applying it to the skin after a bath.

Enteromorpha Intestinalis Elixir

Ingredients:
- 50 g dried enteromorpha intestinalis
- 500 ml alcohol (40-60%, for example vodka)

Preparation: Place the dried Enteromorpha intestinalis in a jar. Cover with alcohol so that the entire seaweed is covered. Close the jar and leave in a dark place for 2-3 weeks, stirring the contents daily. After this time, strain the elixir through a sieve or densely woven cloth, store in a dark bottle.
The Enteromorpha intestinalis elixir has detoxifying and anti-inflammatory properties. It can be used internally (1-2 teaspoons a day) to support digestion and cleanse the body, or externally on the skin to alleviate inflammation and irritation.

Enteromorpha Intestinalis Oil

Ingredients:
- 50 g dried enteromorpha intestinalis
- 500 ml oil (e.g., olive oil, coconut oil)

Preparation: Place the dried Enteromorpha intestinalis in a jar. Pour in the oil so that the entirety is well covered. Close the jar and leave it in a dark, cool place for 4-6 weeks. After this time, strain the oil through a sieve or densely woven cloth, and store it in a dark bottle. The Enteromorpha intestinalis oil acts as a moisturizer and regenerator for the skin. It can be used on all types of skin irritations and inflammations. You can use it like a regular body oil, applying it to the skin after a bath.

Enteromorpha Intestinalis Ointment

Ingredients:

- 1 cup of dried Enteromorpha Intestinalis leaves
- 1/2 cup of coconut oil
- 1/4 cup of beeswax

Preparation: Grind the dried Enteromorpha intestinalis leaves in a coffee grinder or blender to obtain a fine powder. In a small pot, over low heat, melt the coconut oil and beeswax. When the oil and wax are completely melted, add the Enteromorpha intestinalis powder and mix thoroughly. Pour the mixture into a clean jar or other ointment container and let it cool and solidify completely. Store the ointment in a cool, dry place.

This ointment can be applied directly to the skin to help alleviate irritations, prevent infections, and support skin health.

Protein: This seaweed is exceptionally rich in protein, which is necessary for the construction and regeneration of cells in the body.

Vitamins: Enteromorpha intestinalis contains many vitamins, including vitamin C, a powerful antioxidant, and B vitamins, which are necessary for a healthy nervous system.

Minerals: The seaweed is rich in minerals such as iodine, potassium, magnesium, and calcium. These minerals are necessary for the proper functioning of the thyroid, bone and teeth health, proper blood clotting, and maintaining proper blood pressure.

Fiber: Like many other seaweeds, Enteromorpha intestinalis is rich in fiber, which can help maintain a healthy digestive system.

In this chapter, I have brought closer to you the wealth that is the vegetation of our Earth; plants, algae, mosses. These remarkable treasures of nature have been influencing human health for centuries, they are a remedy, they are a discovery, they are a gift. The heritage left to us by the ancient peoples of Europe and the Vikings deserves attention and appreciation. I hand over to you this information, gathered during many hours of studying, noting, and rediscovering.

For nearly 250 pages, I have invited you into a world where medicine and nature go hand in hand, where plants not only heal but also teach us respect for the Earth that offers them. Each page is a fragment of the world that is constantly pulsating with life, giving us resources to care for our body and spirit.

My goal was to show you how connected we are with the Earth, with nature. How much we need these green plants, mosses, algae, which can not only be beautiful elements of our landscape but, above all, an invaluable source of health.

You now know the plants that were used in healing in the past, that helped our ancestors to survive, and today form the basis of many modern medicines.

This chapter is a tribute to nature, to these plants, which in such a wonderful way affect our condition, our mind. They show us how much we should respect this planet, how much we should appreciate what it gives us.

I hope these pages have stimulated you to make a smaller discovery, to reflect on how we live, how we care for our children, how we care for the planet. I am convinced that we have the opportunity to live in harmony with nature, drawing from its benefits, without causing its destruction.

The application of the knowledge of the Vikings and other ancient peoples in practice convinces me that we can become better guardians of our planet.

Modern times focus on profit, often neglecting an ecological lifestyle and harmonious coexistence with nature, as well as concern for the health of our planet. We should already start taking daily actions that will help keep our planet in an immaculate state.

During walks in the forest, park, or coastline, we should appreciate its primal, undisturbed form. It is in these distant corners of the Earth, where man has not yet left his destructive mark, where grow extraordinary plants not only beautiful but also beneficial for our health, our journey towards health and harmony with the natural world begins.

But I would like to emphasize one thing. We must not treat these places as sources of infinite resources. Just because nature offers us such wealth does not mean that we can use it without moderation.

Therefore, my priority is to ensure that the use of medicinal plants, mosses, algae takes place with respect for nature.

Collection should be responsible, with respect for the plants and the environment in which they grow.

When collecting, remember not to destroy plants, not to tear them out with their roots, not to take too many specimens, to remember to preserve species diversity. Remember that plants are not just a collection of medicines, but true organisms that have their place in the ecosystem. They are home to many species of animals, they clean the air we breathe, they hold water in the soil, preventing erosion. Without them, our planet would not be as it is today.

I would like this chapter to inspire you, Dear Reader, to reflect on your own relationship with nature. To understand how important it is to find a balance between benefiting from the bounties of the earth and caring for its survival.

We can draw from it, but we must also give, care, protect. Therefore, let the knowledge that I have passed on to you serve not only to improve your health but also to deepen your understanding and respect for our planet.

The adventure with nature, with its herbs, plants, and marine algae is not only a path to improve our health but also to a deeper understanding of the world in which we live. Each plant we get to know reminds us of the incredible diversity of life on Earth and how important it is to protect it.

When we gather herbs or algae, we learn to observe, appreciate, and respect life in every form.

We also learn that nature is our greatest teacher - each plant, each animal has some lesson to impart.

By discovering the application of plants in medicine, we can understand how much we depend on the health of our planet. Therefore, when you benefit from the bounties of nature, remember your responsibility.

Take care of biodiversity, cleanse the environment, protect and help plants and animals. Take care of harmony with nature, because it is our home, our heritage, which we have a duty to pass on to future generations.

May the knowledge that I have passed on to you become a guidepost for you. May it lead you to a healthier life, to harmony with nature, and to a fuller understanding of how valuable our planet is.

May it inspire you to further search, to learn, and to discover.

Because each of us has the potential to become a guardian of the Earth, to protect and nurture its beauty for future generations.

We have just completed our journey through the fascinating world of natural medicine, discovering together the remarkable medicinal properties of many plants.

I hope our virtual expedition has opened new horizons for you and now, when you go for a walk, you will happily notice these wonderful plants that surround us everywhere in our daily lives.

Remember, each of these plants is not just a pretty decoration of nature, but real health treasures, full of wealth that humans have been utilizing since the earliest times. Some of them have accompanied us for centuries, constituting a key element of our ancestors' tradition and culture, others we are only discovering now, thanks to the progress of science and pharmacy.

The next time you see, for example, a bog-rosemary, think about its extraordinary properties, about the people who discovered its power centuries ago, and also about how it is now used in modern medicine.

This approach will allow you to look at the world of plants from a completely new perspective. Soon we will embark on another journey together, where I will be happy to help you discover even more treasures that our magnificent planet offers us.

See you on the next walk, full of discoveries and fascinating stories!

Your Herbal Cultivation and Harvest Table

Pos.	Planting Time	Planting Location	Harvest Time	Harvest Place	Drying Temp

ABOUT THE AUTHOR

The author of „The Berserker's Gardens and Forests" is a person with many passions, but above all deeply rooted in love for nature.

He has spent many years studying the cultural heritage of the Vikings and ancient peoples of Europe, their understanding of nature and ways of using plants in healing and everyday life. He is not only a researcher and scholar, but also a practitioner.

He enthusiastically uses the gifts of nature in his daily life, convinced of their extraordinary health potential.

In his work, he strives to discover and convey this invaluable knowledge, hoping to improve the quality of life for readers. His beliefs and aspirations are consistent with the philosophy of sustainable development.

He believes that we can draw from the Earth's bounty while caring for its protection and survival. That's why in his book, he emphasizes the importance of harmonious coexistence with nature and respect for its gifts.

He is also deeply engaged in promoting a healthy lifestyle and natural medicine, and „The Berserker's Gardens and Forests" is an expression of this commitment - a book written with passion, knowledge and conviction that everyone can benefit from a closer contact with nature.

INSPIRED BY THE WEALTH OF NATURE

www.eco-loco.life

Table of Contents

SPECIAL THANKS TO STUDIO KREATYWNE KAROLINA WIETESKA A FOR GRAPHIC AND TECHNICAL SUPPORT

Made in United States
Orlando, FL
04 November 2026

90201355R00155